FROM THE INSIDE

A Look at Nursing Homes and Their Patients in Todays Elder Care System

June A. W. Severance

June A. W. Severance

Copyright © 2012 by June A. W. Severance

Edited by Mary Ann Peck.
Cover design by Larry Addington, 20/20 Designs, Ashland, OR.

ISBN: Paperback   978-0-9851102-2-2
ISBN-10:   0985110228

Although all names of persons and places have been changed, the
incidents portray the author's real experiences.

This book was printed in the United States of America.

Additional copies may be ordered from:

Amazon.com

and

peckpublishing.org

June A. W. Severance

TABLE OF CONTENTS

PART I

June A. W. Severance

PART II

Beloved Life Stories

Fred

Bert

Madeline

Helen

The Seraphim & Cherubim

Altha Mae

Edith

The Cowboy

Harold & Ellie

Rose

Edwina

Sand Dollars

My Last Roommate

Departures and Goodbyes

June A. W. Severance

APPENDIX

Resident's Rights

State and Federal Regulations
http://www.hpm.umn.edu/nhregsplus/NH%20Regs%20by%20Topic/NH%20Regs%20Topic%20Pdfs/Resident%20Rights/category_resident_rights_FINAL.pdf

DEDICATION

To my husband, Wayne, who sustains me
as Browning says:

Grow old with me,
  the best is yet to be.
The last of life for which
  the first was made.

To Jennifer Andren who felt/knew the
meaning as she typed the manuscript.

June A. W. Severance

PART I

Introduction

June A. W. Severance

Introduction to a Nursing Home

The Admissions Director was a jolly cheerleader type and asked, "What are your father's hobbies?"

"Well, he hasn't been able to do much..."

"Oh, I mean what are his interests. I'm fitting him with a roommate. Be great to have him with someone who has the same likes, you know!" She shuffled papers, smiling. She was a bouncy lady.

Was I filling out applications for my 78 year-old father to go to summer camp or to enroll in college as a beanie-wearing freshman? I lamely thought up something.

"Long ago he could speak some German and..."

"Cool! There's just the roomie! Speaks German and..."

I hated to jump up but I wanted to get out of this 'cool' place without delay.

"The records from the hospital must show that Dad can't speak at all....aphasia..." I was furious.

Three years before, Dad and Mother had moved in with me, my husband and our sons. When Mother decided Dad should go into a nursing home, I had to relent. So there I was, wasting time with this 'frisky' lady while an ambulance was on the way to this facility, transporting my father from the hospital.

Was she ever going to review Dad's case and simply get him a bed? No, first the paperwork, then the walk-through of this Nursing Home, Miami Beach Hotel perfect! The folks groggily lounging in a row along the walls of the great room/living room— whatever the label—more like Florida snowbirds, were probably talking about their bodily functions. If I'd been closer to them, I'd have seen they were not talking at all, nor was anyone talking to them.

Finally, my father was assigned a room with a glum gentleman. Aides flitted in and out. I was so negative about his being there I could only see him being curtly wheeled out into the hall for lunch and dinner and then moved about to get him out of the way, when the vacuuming person came down the hall..

The nursing home 'jolly time' concluded with my father's return to the hospital. He contracted pneumonia after being left in front of an open window.

Due to my father's skilled nursing home experience, my prejudices, truly pre-judgments were there years later, when it was my turn.

I also would have a near-death experience due to an oversight; however, I learned the good along with the not-so-good *FROM THE INSIDE.*[1]

---

[1] Guide to Choosing a Nursing Home
http://www.medicare.gov/Library/PDFNavigation/PDFInterim.asp?Language=English&Type=Pub&PubID=02174

Chapter I

My First Days

My life *FROM THE INSIDE* began when I arrived by ambulance at the nursing home on a spring evening. Late sunglow was on the trees outside the beautifully dressed windows -- three wide, wonderful windows. A male attendant gave me fresh hospital nightwear with ties in the back and a crisp, striped robe that closed in the front. I remember most his bringing out toothbrushes and asking my favorite color.

"Blue," I answered.

"I found a blue one for you!"

Somehow, as I moved from the commode into bed, his holding up the blue one put me at peace. I settled in the bed, letting the pain sink under the covers and turned to the pink afterglow on the trees I saw from the lovely windows.

"How did you fall and break your hip?" one of the Aides asked me the next day.

"I had a total hip replacement."

"Oh, you're post-surgery. Usually the other hip has to be replaced," said the other Aide.

Above my head were instructions in boldface print and the extent of the movements. "NO crossing the involved leg more than forty-five degrees."

Then, on bright orange construction paper, was the "List of Meds" posted by a young, serious Aide whom I saw only once. She gave me a plastic

container with little cramped sections for each day --
a.m., noon, midday, bedtime. The column for Sunday
was missing. She noted this but never returned, a most
mysterious young woman.

Other Aides stopped in during the night, and as
time passed, they became my beloveds. One, a large
Native American young man, was the one who held
me as I sobbed when a violent pain persisted, not in
the new hip joint, but a large blood clot in a lung.
Another Aide, who ran a private religious school by
day, wracked his brain to help me, using his Army
Medical Corp training.

"We'll try big pillows behind you."

However, in physical therapy, the director
disregarded even my tears, and went on with the
exercises. One day she said, "We have an example of
'cry wolf' perhaps."

During the many weeks of P.T. room workouts,
I had cried once or twice foolishly, not primarily from
pain but being tired and over-stimulated. My
roommate's daughters brought food to her at midnight
and stayed to talk together for hours.

One daughter preached exotic foods, and told
me my inner turmoil would result in heart trouble. The
power of the mind, challenging mind! Perhaps this was
her logic, but she should not have been allowed to
mesmerize me at two and three a.m. I never thought I
would have heart trouble.

There was good and bad inside a nursing home.
The discipline for patients not bed-ridden was
excellent. Pre-breakfast routine was good for me. I
moved into a wheelchair and rolled over to the sink for

self wash-up. Then I wheeled over to a closet and
chose the day's ensemble -- actually any nicely printed,
open-in-the-back frock. I learned to push my arms
into the sleeves, flip the cloth over legs and around the
back, and even to button or tie the garment. Heaven
forbid I might tip out of the chair! Quite revealing! I
enjoyed being ready for the assigned dining room. It
was part of the big Day Room, which had beautiful
decor and more large windows. Here, the more able
patients ate at what I soon called the *Directors'* table.
Smiling Fred B, white haired, dignified, perfect CEO,
President of the Board had his wheelchair placed at the
head of the table.

Various glum, shy, tentative folk were on either
side. Norma from California, M.T. an artist and I were
at the far end. Meals were full of conversation!

Norma's tone was bitter, tight, Hollywood wit—
much about a grandson in films and her son moving
her to this small city because he was having an
apartment built onto his home. She described the size
and the gorgeous grounds, where she would soon be
living.

"I won't be living in this jail," she said.

I learned Norma would be stabilized. She
needed physical movement, which she refused to do,
and therefore continued to weaken. Digestive
problems required special food regimen, which she
also refused. I was drawn to Norma, her rage, her
fine-boned face, the obsidian eyes. Her drawl had
remnants of her Texas youth, although she had been
living in California for decades.

"My son took training for machine work and moved up in my company." Norma felt superior to the limp patients she feared becoming.

"What good am I now?" she blurted as she told me about her two devastating strokes.

"They've taken away half my body!" she continued, adding a few earthy 'damns!'

I told her I would storm the Gates of Heaven so that she could walk again and I would persist because I wanted to know her better.

The situation was different when Olivia was wheeled to our table. Getting-to-know-her was not my desire. She was an "I" person—quite lofty. Townspeople who knew Olivia gossiped, "Her CEO husband died to get away from her."

Olivia declared, "I'll be going to my card clubs. The facility van will take me every Wednesday. Right after breakfast, I will be taken to the beautician." She was chagrined to learn the facility's hairdresser was not there every day!

M.T. would flicker amused eye signals at me. Fred B. mediated when a few folks at our table were glum, especially one gentleman whose wife loyally came to help him at mealtimes, but he seldom said a word to her or to us.

After breakfast, the medicine woman tapped me on the shoulder. She pushed a big multi-tiered cart which had little paper cups. Was she arranging a children's party? Patients were handed these cups and some were expected to swallow these pills with applesauce. I was in awe of her knowledge. She dispensed meds under strict parameters. She carried a photo of each patient and their list of dosages. After testing me on her explanation of my meds, she said I had to identify each one. Two were yellow, but one was smaller, so I guessed correctly.

"But how do they know where to go?" I wanted to ask. Instead, a picture came to my mind of the medicine catapulting down my esophagus in panic! The medicine woman would not want this idle puzzlement. She had many to help, so off she went.

In addition, I will always remember the funniest morning. Everyone at our *Board of Directors* table was flip-flapping fried eggs on the plates. Even gracious Fred was pushing them around, saying, "Rubber! That's what these are!"

The dietician arrived at our table and explained how she had orders from the new health department inspector to avoid salmonella poisoning by cooking eggs at high temperatures.

Norma spat out, "I'd rather have salmonella!"

"No you wouldn't!" I retorted.

Norma ate so little and complained so much that her fury did not impress me. We had good rapport so could be bold with each other. I could nag her to eat, saying she needed to get strong enough if she wants to get out!

The rubber food was taken away. There was peace, toast and tea.

After breakfast, but before morning physical therapy, I enjoyed wheeling beside M.T. as she walked slowly, leaning on her high walker. She had metal braces on her legs. M.T. never explained her disabilities, but when I went to her room, I was dismayed at the swarm of medical bills. They spilled over her bedside table and her artwork supplies. I liked looking at her exquisite paintings. Flowers blossomed directly out of her canvases!

Mid-morning, we went to P.T., deemed by many people as the best department in the facility.

Chapter II

P.T. and O.T.

Physical therapy, both morning and afternoon, began with stretching exercises. Those who could stand, worked at a support bar, others like me worked diligently from wheelchairs.

Leg weights made the workout more intense, especially when I lay flat on a low leather bed provided for those who could not lie on a floor mat. Later, I tried the challenging stair steps one riser at a time, then still later awkwardly with a walker.

The arm or leg movements were vigorous, with many 'reps' as repeats were called. The work was exact if the therapist was precise, a bit casual if directed by a P.T Aide in training. Still it was good stimulation and self-discipline that I needed. I worked hard despite pain, and secretly agreed with the hot-tempered Director of P.T. when she said of me, "She could teach the course; she's memorized the routine!"

In her mercurial way, the Director was wishing I would be discharged. Some personalities do conflict, as she and I did. Her compliment was given at an assessment conference. The other staff was concerned because I lived a long distance from the nursing home.

Two directors had driven the 120 miles to advise about my post-rehabilitation needs: width of doorways, height of chairs, ramps to be built. However, I had not practiced with a walker nor worked in occupational therapy (O.T.) to be able to manage daily tasks at home, e.g. cooking. The nursing home had a complete kitchen, a workshop for crafts, and a small greenhouse, which were all stimulating, excellent places and kept patients moving. My first O.T. experiences were in the kitchen where, unfortunately, sporadic attention occurred. I was a whiz cutting up strawberries, but baking a cake was a challenge as I rose from my wheelchair, leaned on a walker, and flayed away with a 'grabber'—a device used in grocery stores to get items placed on high shelves. The handle squeezes two long pieces of springy metal curved at the ends, where two suction cups come together to grab anything rubber can. Plump Benjamin Franklin invented this device to avoid climbing a ladder to reach his books. It gives one an extra arm's length for reaching grandchildren, too!

However, an egg is most illusive, and I was totally defeated by cantaloupe. Most items in a refrigerator slyly retreat to the back of the shelf when pursued; same problem with an oven rack. I had a smaller device to aid me: a wooden stick with a tiny rubber hook which melted in the oven when I tried to bring out a rack.

I went on the wild quest for measuring cups, spices, and sugars in the low drawers of the practice kitchen. The Aide for this O.T. cake assignment had dissolved down the hall after having airily pointed to the counters and cupboards where I was to find everything needed to make the cake. Bowls I could reach and proper pans were also deep within the drawers, which I could open by clutching the kitchen counter as I pulled on the handles. I finally had the batter ready and poured, oh, so slowly and shakily, into pans, but there were no knobs on the oven. How was I to bake this blasted batter? This was the great idea to prepare patients for daily living. Here was a rare example of total employee failure. I longed to give up, just to retreat to bed if I had been able to transfer myself from my wheelchair.

Finally, a different Aide appeared. She showed me how the magic oven was controlled by a switch high on the wall around the corner from the stove. To prevent disoriented patients from turning them on, all the stove's knobs were there, unmarked. As I left that area, I realized it was not far from the dining room for the severely afflicted stroke and Alzheimer's patients. There, I saw the compassionate Aides feeding and calming the helpless—making my frustrations quite petulant. We complain about our shoes and then we see human beings without feet. The cake was baked and used at a happy time we will learn about later.

June A. W. Severance

Chapter III

Conditioned Response

No, we are not Pavlov's dogs[2], although his experiment led to an understanding —our reactions to repeated stimuli don't always reach agreement.

In a 2008 spring issue of AARP[3], there appeared a report of a disabled man fighting Florida's mandate that he must live in a nursing home. He feared the

---

[2] Classical conditioning (also Pavlovian conditioning or respondent conditioning) is a form of learning in which one stimulus, the *conditioned stimulus* or CS, comes to signal the occurrence of a second stimulus, the *unconditioned stimulus* or US. The US is usually a biologically significant stimulus such as food or pain that elicits a response from the start; this is called the *unconditioned response* or UR. The CS usually produces no particular response at first, but after conditioning it elicits the *conditioned response* or CR. Classical conditioning differs from *operant or instrumental conditioning*, in which behavior emitted by the organism is strengthened or weakened by its consequences, e.g. reward or punishment.

[3] American Association of Retired Persons

forced scheduling of his life with his days planned for him. He hinted he might become like other paraplegics and become accustomed, even perhaps develop an *accommodation expectation.*

Nursing home conditioning or scheduling the patient's life, gives habits to which he/she becomes habituated. I experienced this even in a stay of only six months.

As my pragmatic, wise mother-in-law said, "Gets so you can't change. It's all in what you're used to." She was speaking of general living: it's more true in an institution.

A New York State Supreme Court Judge I knew was a feisty man. He was a challenge and a delight to be around. He'd been a 'fair-haired' lad in his Irish neighborhood because he had a withered leg from early childhood polio. His crutches were simply a part of his body and with them, he made his way to the nearby swimming hole, or to jobs, onto buses to his college and law school campus refusing a lift as cars came along the road. Oh, he also played golf and a mean game of ping-pong with his seven offspring. I was hired as a companion and reader when the Judge's failing eyesight compelled him to step down from the bench. To me, he was a bit of a leprechaun with his own brand of magic.

After the Judge had to be placed in a skilled nursing home, I asked his wife when I could visit him. Margaret was gracious and usually a cheerful woman who was devoted to the Judge. Now she answered sadly.

"It's only been a short time, but he's a different man. Not our Judge. You don't want to see him this way."

I could remember his constant way of teasing as he came to meet me at his front door. The crutches were always tucked under his armpits, and he would rub his hands together. "And what is on the agenda for today, Mrs. S?"

The Judge's eyes would sparkle. He disliked regimentation or even the hint of it. Did the routine, the necessary rules of the institution numb him? He was not obstreperous, like the Rose of my poem. Did his spirit break under the loss of his prestigious position in the court and as an autocrat-at-the-breakfast table at home? Did he feel confined, having been accustomed to a large home, despite the spacious gathering rooms of the nursing facility? Being regarded as frail, and dependent enough to have to be in a skilled nursing home, seemed to have dissolved the Judge. He no longer smiled nor responded. I was shocked! He let everyone go past him without a greeting. Staff just led him along.

The other side to 'conditioning' occurs when a patient becomes contented. A friend of mine was in rehabilitation after war injuries, and he told me, "I was a changed person. I had good care and I became used to people around me, all doing things together. I got too used to being in an institution where I was safe. I became afraid to try any other world."

Yes, whether you are in for a short time or a long period, what you become used to can lead to a phenomenon called 'obedience'. Yes, it is necessary to have rules, but some patients become too docile and lose initiative. Hence, a typical scene viewed from the outside of 'old folks in the home' just sitting, napping in a row of chairs. Is this numbness a result of being caught up in the routine, necessary as it is, of group living?

Perhaps concern over being on time for scheduled meals and for medical treatments has a limiting effect on patients. We all know the stifling of incentive, our own dismissing the urge we felt to begin an activity. If we do this to ourselves, how easy it is to stifle our own initiative when daily life is planned for us. How do we go from a lifetime of adventure to non-adventure? It is also a chicken-and-the-egg dilemma: do weeks in routine diminish activity even with scheduled events having been designed for activity? No, what occurs is dependence; becoming used to having decisions made for us. Meals become occasions to be on time.

You can see a line of nursing home clients moving towards the dining area long ahead of schedule, sometimes at the expense of a visitor who had 'dropped in'. They anxiously look forward to see if fellow inmates are heading for Craft Time, Exercise, and Snack Time. Obedience curtails spontaneity.

There are poignant examples. My elderly aunt lived in a crowded, rather unpleasant, nursing home that did manage to shut out the noisy rush of traffic and the dangers of her city. Our visits to Aunt Jean began with her flashing smiles. We did not flinch as her dentures became ugly and she was failing. We enjoyed being with the Jean, whom we loved and wanted to make the most of our time. Soon she looked toward the hallway asking, "Where's Sally? We must call her to come here."

While we, the real family of Jean's 90-plus years, were happy that she had Sally as a close daily companion, we did not make the trip from out of town to see Sally. In addition, we could see Jean's eyes dismissing us--not rudely--oh no. We understood and knew the nursing home was now, truly, Jean's world.

We disengaged our hearts, feeling the wrench, and learned what one daily endures becomes their world. Conditioning took over -- for us, too.

Another example: a charming couple we had socialized with in our town for over a decade. The man had battled leukemia but went to work every day even though he had a long commute. He had times of remission, then flare-ups, and recently a broken hip. He truly declared himself a 'survivor!' Vigorous physical therapy had him walking again with a walker, and he still declared, "I'm kept on this earth to take care of this kid!"

The "kid" is actually many calendar years older, but to him and to us, she is ageless, a sparkling old beauty! This gal has had countless careers from rough Chicago real estate, running a dance studio, flying planes, cooking for her own restaurant, and managing a Los Angeles music store. Now she chuckles over most of the statements we make, her eyes gleaming with a clever cover-up if the given day is not the most lucid. She recovered from strokes and T.I.A.'s. "Very clearly," she said, as I sat beside her in their rest home's lovely dining room, "I'm enjoying life."

This couple enjoys outings with us, and being helped into a car to attend church. However, as we have spent time together, we have seen a subtle change enveloping them. They repeat things such as the time we must return; their eyes are on the clock. We are joyful that all goes well in their skilled nursing home, but we see them being pulled to the schedule and to their new families -- the conditioned response again. Outsiders like us now observe the change in their interactions: clients are more spontaneous with their daily contacts on the inside.

Example: the day nurse comes into their room. She smiles. Smiles beam back to her and the conversation turns to -- "That's a new blouse! Looks so pretty, Sarah! Oh, we ordered your favorite kind of potatoes for the cook to make! Don't forget, tomorrow's bath day!"

It is human nature. Visitors keep telling themselves they should visit the home. Nevertheless, the twinges of guilt subside when the patients turn them off.

"Oh, Wednesday? No, there's Exercise class and after that, I am usually tired. Maybe you can come another day."

Alternatively, "Oh, that's the same afternoon we have Bingo. Next Tuesday? A lady comes to read to us and then we play cards."

I began to wonder how I reacted as a patient. I had written before of my despair -- the pain was affecting me so much I could only relate to and depend on the nursing staff. I even thought only they could 'deal' with me. My former existence of being a theater director, daily news commentator on radio, even the more recent work of my town's publicity project—all became alien and part of the 'outside'. To muster up confidence and decisiveness seemed impossible and even frightening. The pain began the process. I was becoming comfortable with life 'inside' and I was less aware of the outside world's events.

Propinquity—comfort in the immediate people, staff and fellow patients. I was happy to see their faces by day and night. I tried to bridge the two worlds, but I was dangerously close to retreating into my daily conditioning. I was too safe in the nursing home.

June A. W. Severance

Chapter IV

Critic to Suzy-Camper Activities

One of the areas I came to know changed my pre-judgments about nursing homes. I understood the planning and the psychology involved with activities I once scorned as 'cutesy.' Even with the burden of aphasia, speech-mind connection, my Dad's hands were efficient, as well as his eyesight. Perhaps I could have helped him by learning the skills of the Craft Director as I observed patients doing scrap booking. He did not need speech. Dad could listen and make sense of directions.

When I was on the inside, I first was interested in the little greenhouse and became Suzy-camper as I bid my husband goodbye. "I'm fine! I'm going to plant things with my friend MT, she's a master-gardener."

Yes, encouraged by the Activity Director, MT manipulated a long hoe from her high walker nestling seedlings into the outside soil. In the greenhouse, we both worked from wheelchairs we had drawn up to tables. The Activity Director impressed me. She was precise. Tasks were well organized. She joked that she was trained in Germany and that's how we had to be! I asked where in Germany, and she thought I would not know the town at the confluence of the Rhine and the Moselle....

"My great-grandmother came from Coblenz-in-the-Moselle. She always insisted on saying the full name." I babbled.

"Ach! My town!" We both lit up with delight. "I'll bring photos."

We soon were instructed in sand play; well, actually, layers of colored sand we arranged in glass containers instead of on the ground like Tibetan sand wheels.

The colors we chose were symbolic of our wishes. We put them in order of priority while enjoying the tactile sensation of sand sliding through our fists. I picked blue for the sky and visions therein; light blue and dark. Gold tones for sun and joy, orange-rust of lichen, symbiotic with boulders I like. Busy with my hands, I didn't worry about pain. Then having the beauty of something I made cheered me.

See, we scorn and then stay to pray. How I had misunderstood the point of disabled patients toddling to a craft room of nursing homes I had visited. I only saw the green-ware, silly frogs or curved vases that few people wanted. In "Happy Hollow" or "Sunny Castle" rest homes, I saw patients who no longer owned cars or homes requiring keys, all busy making key chains. Yes, it was easy for me, for any of us, to spurn until we walk in another person's moccasins. The key chains would make gifts for a patient's family and friends and were a source of creative accomplishment.

I also had not realized the importance of what I regarded as jolly notices on the bulletin boards of the homes. The calendars were filled with card-playing schedules, dates of birthdays, and the parties. There is a need for the posted name and numerical date of each day as well as the season and the weather outside. In the world of any institution, patients can lose awareness of the outer world. Much care goes into those calendars on the bulletin boards as well as the holiday decorations, the musical and inspirational programs. Local church groups make regular visits; priests and ministers bring religious services right into the nursing homes. These comforting activities are all listed, and Aides help patients notice what they can look forward to in the well-run nursing homes.

The bulletin board has the important hotline of the state ombudsman who addresses patient grievances. Monthly meetings of the resident council and the community-family council are listed. Patients elect the head of their resident group, who must be proud to see his/her name on the calendars of their meetings.

June A. W. Severance

Chapter V

Contrasts

She said her name was Jennie Virginia Mabel…
"Whoa!" I said. "So many names!"

The pretty, silver-haired woman laughed, "Why, yes, mother was so glad to have a girl finally, she used all the girly names on her list."

I looked from my wheelchair to hers. Jennie's merry eyes hinted she was teasing all of us gathered in the gazebo on a sunny afternoon. She had not been one of the O.T. skills group cutting up strawberries the day before when I had my cake-baking adventure. Now we were able to get acquainted at a tea party arranged by the staff. We were surrounded by beautiful flowers chosen by M.T. and the couple who played violin and piano. That day we all relaxed, forgot leg braces and pain. The violin lady wowed us about her husband's having been a Prohibition "rum-runner" on the North Dakota-Canadian border.

I made sure to visit with Jennie-of-the-many-names after the tea party. She was proud of the grandson who came frequently to help her practice on her walker. He was on a school board, a real leader in his town.

"And you grew up there?" I asked.

"No, I was raised way up in the mountains." Jennie explained. "Dad found a place that was proved up and someone to work it. Mother and he farmed back in Kansas, saved, raised up fine boys. Then when the oldest were good ages to help, eight and nine, Dad put everything in a wagon and came out here. How the boys crowed when I was born! A girl to do the inside chores! But I liked being outdoors. Could ride my little horse better than any of them. One time I chased them all the way to my uncle's ranch. I knew they were going up in the mountains to drive the sheep to summer pasture... Maybe stay for weeks even!"

"Were you sent home?" I asked.

"No, my aunt understood and my uncle sent one of the boys home for my camp clothes. I was in double trouble. I'd jumped on my horse in my best pinafore; mamma liked a girl to look nice. I went up with them and slept in a Sougan, saw the Shining Mountains close up."

"Was there always your family on Sheep Creek?"

"Not at first. Mother didn't see another white woman in the first two years. Squaws would come up, wait so quiet and then just walk in the back door. Used to that, I guess, no doors to knock on in teepees. They taught mamma how to dry their kind of squashes and how to make pemmican. The men showed Dad the best wild grasses. Our stock really thrived."

"Did your mother find it hard, just being there alone?"

"No. We went to town now and again. Sold what we grew in the nearest town. Then, near Christmas time, we'd take the train all the way to a big city. Oh, that was special, and cold! We kids were bundled up in the wagon to get to the train station and back. The boys rolled us up in Sougans; guess they used the horse blankets. I remember we would just have the tips of our noses out. We'd push up just a minute to see the stars. Oh, how they glittered!"

One day later, Jennie announced, "I'm going home tomorrow!" We'd met in the hall, Jennie using the walker, standing so straight as she walked the length of our wing, a long hallway.

"Home! I'm glad for you Jennie. Home to the ranch?"

"No, in town."

I remembered she'd mentioned all the grand and great-grands living just blocks from each other—all near her. Her brothers had sold the big ranch to an out-of-stater who hired her nephew as manager.

"The owner's a young man and he likes it up there. Does not know a thing about ranching. Thank goodness, my Lowell lives right on the place. The new fellow didn't even know how to open a hay bale."

"Twine's pretty complicated!" We laughed together.

"He wanted to buy up loads of just alfalfa for his new horses that would have done them in! Too hot. Our Lowell put him straight; he's a fine rancher." Such pride in Jennie's voice, Jennie the fine lady, waving as she went home, healed.

Throughout Jerry Freedman's book, *Earth's Elders*, he described folks living past one-hundred thriving best with family links on a daily basis. My friend Virginia glowed as her grandson and his family escorted her to their car. She had described how her school-age great-grandchildren ran to hug her as they came home from school. "Dropped those backpacks and called out 'How are you today gram-gram?'"

Compared with Virginia, Jenny, etc., Norma would seem a glaring contrast. From California, she dressed in correct and sophisticated outfits even to the right earrings. The Aides loved dressing her.

After some strokes, Norma was brought to this Nursing Home-Rehab located near her eldest son.

"I'm not staying here – he has a big spread and he's building an apartment for me!"

Norma's obsidian eyes would close as her handsome face turned away. She was bitter that the strokes did not let her complete a sentence or a witty anecdote. At our special table, Norma pushed her wheelchair away with her graceful hands. "Tell you, other time."

She tolerated my nagging to remain and eat more to get stronger.

"Not this pap! I know you – smart one." Her smile belied her anger.

I could feel the wit even unspoken and later learned she raised her three sons alone, having dumped a dull husband. She worked in a war plant, "Moved up. Needed smart women in World War II."

As years went by, I visited a bright, vociferous Norma. I worried that her family was stringing her along. A relative took me aside, explaining that Norma was never going to live at the big house in a mythical apartment. Though Norma called it jail, she was to remain at the nursing home. Our visits became full of affection and shared gossip about patients and especially the Aides. She liked one who brought his ever-increasing flock of children to see Norma. She cooed over how movie hero handsome he was.

"Now come in my room and we can really talk about Hollywood." We looked at all the photos on her wall. "My middle son just barged in the studio lot and got a job in the stables. John Wayne noticed his spunk, put him, you know, in touch with some big shots. Just think, he's lived his dream of a career in films! That latest picture, see, he sent me from where he's on location in Spain."

"Norma, seems like he has his mother's spunk."

Her old Texas twang rolled with that. "Yes, worked my way up to supervisor in that war plant, raised my kids like I planned in California. I moved there from a dirt-poor town in Texas."

She described recent dinners with her family at the area's best restaurants. "Great weekends. Went to the mall – had to be sure the oldest granddaughter picked out the right prom dress."

One October day Norma was excited. She had bought a costume for the Nursing Home's Halloween Party. "Mine'll be the best one here."

Oh yes, the overnight visits to her son's home were nice but even at Thanksgiving she came back to the Nursing Home early.

"Funny to say, but I'm eager to get peaceful here. Oh, they're all fun. But back here, I'm cozy and, you know, my roommate is so sweet."

What a switch!

June A. W. Severance

Chapter VI

Couples Hand in Hand

From "Residents Rights"[4] the right to share a room with your spouse living in the same facility. Hence, a couple in another nursing home shared a large unit with a kitchen and divider wall between it and the bedroom.

They joined other residents for major meals. The husband kept up with the town library's Book Club, and both went to church, transported by the facility's van, which took residents to medical appointments and to visit if one spouse was hospitalized. This excellent service at my nursing home also eased worry and hastened recovery.

A beautiful cut-out of a violin decorated the door of a room belonging to a couple who rehearsed there for weekly programs of violin and piano.

I was awed by their music, knowing they both dealt with illness. They did not stop bringing joy and

---

[4] See Appendix or Patient's Rights online – appendix page 116.
http://www.nationalhealthcouncil.org/pages/page-content.php?pageid=66

delighted in Saturday afternoon movies in the Day Room where the staff even brought a popcorn machine. The couple held hands during love scenes.

Another couple, not sharing a room but always together, tugged at my heart. When I first shook hands with Steve, he was newly confined to a wheel chair, and able to sit up straight, very straight and full of a young man's fury. As years went by, Steve railed against his devastating disability; I did not inquire, as that would have gone against *Residents Right of Confidentiality*. He eventually could hardly retain our handshake and only sprawled in his wheelchair. When I visited from the Outside, I hoped Steve did not resent me; but as our eyes really communicated, he relaxed. I knew he accepted my concern and he did not have to talk, for any sentiment was directed and shared with blonde, pretty Claire, who was under the guardianship of the state. There were a few other clients in our home in the same position.

"Steve" and "Claire" -- need linked to need. She stayed beside him, pushed the wheelchair, helped him eat, gentle with him when he sometimes threw his plate on the floor. Her arm would go around his tense, surly shoulders and in corners they would kiss. She wheeled him to the home's live entertainment programs and to the movies. Claire had a reason to live and Steve, a reason not to die too soon.

A woman I came to know in another skilled nursing facility was likewise loved by her mate who took an apartment nearby and spent the time remaining for them with this always smiling invalid. Her muscles were slowly atrophying, no cure. She made exquisite decorations, attaching sequins and pearl beads to styrofoam forms. Her hands were open to everyone.

She gave away these bright, sparkling creations made with her still flexible hands as she sat strapped to her chair with her husband beside her.

June A. W. Severance

Chapter VII

Days toward the Crisis and Beyond

"WHY?" I wrote. The arresting word was all I could think, when the mysterious PAIN added to the daily pain.

"Why was I still alive?"

I learned later that more than normal blood remained in the "pocket" at my new hip joint. One or more clots formed in the weeks of healing, absolutely contrary to medical theory.

I was working diligently on the physical therapy exercises, moving both the 'involved' leg and the other leg. I had flexed and waved legs in the air, walked the treadmill, rotated ankles when in bed, pedal-paddled my feet on the floor as I rolled my wheelchair.

Still pain, constantly sharp wires, went through me as I stood, took steps and leaned on the walker. Afterward as I breathed deep came excruciating, sharp stabs. Oh, I seemed such a wimp. I was helped when an infected tooth set me crying. Aides brought flexible rice packs[5] heated in the microwave.

Theories abounded. Had tube breathing in my mouth after surgery injured my mouth or jaw? No. All was settled by a trip to a local dentist who willingly worked on me, bending down to the wheelchair. No way could I be helped up onto the regular dental chair, which would have been much easier for him[6]. He removed the infected tooth.

While I struggled with PAIN, I wrote: "When the body becomes alien, unpredictable, a body one cannot depend on, does one then pull away from familiar people? Even flinch from being back home? Not being as I once was, do I not want to be with people who do not know this alien being? Do I think only the people in the medical world can deal with me now?"

---

[5] http://www.ehow.com/how_7698682_directions-make-rice-packs.html *Rice* can be sewn into pieces of cloth to make a compress or pillow-type pack. These can be put into the freezer for cold applications such as sprains or aches, or microwaved to create a hot pillow similar to a hot-water bottle for achy muscles. Scents can be added to the pillow during the sewing process through the use of essential oils or herbs. The packs can be further customized through the use of various types of materials, colors and patterns.

[6] Medically interesting: *a year later this very intelligent DDS attended a conference about causal relationship between tooth infections and heart and lung complications.*

Such thinking is an example of the conditioning noted in nursing home patients. It is a form of dependence.[7]

Then the words I wrote in a very different and shaky hand one midnight: IT BURNS—I WISH MY CHEST WOULD EXPLODE OR I COULD DIE.

I do remember wanting to smash the walker into the room's big picture window, but then my practical side held me back.

"You don't destroy property nor make a mess," I told myself.

The fury did explode in sobbing. I hated to be so noisy that I woke my roommate, but I could not stop the hysterical crying. I could only claw at the strong hands of the Aide, Ryan, who had come to help me late that night.

An alert R.N. waylaid a doctor making his rounds in the nursing home. This R.N. noticed I had changed. She said I was no longer trying to do things for myself. I actually drooped in my wheelchair. I remember staring at the hall carpet wishing I could disappear into it.

X-rays showed something in the right lung. Yes, the pain shot through that side. Why hadn't the head physical therapist believed me? Then the Doppler machine, ultrasound, showed the vivid picture—a big thing in the leg—and another like a grub in a tunnel (my words). Embolisms. A near-fatal second blood clot had gone to a lung.

---

[7] See Chapter III, Conditioned Response

"Six hours to live!" the doctors told me. That is, if I would lie flat on my back with minimal motion. That's what I did, beyond the crisis, for seven days back in the hospital. Blessed respiratory therapists administered medicine by means of a nebulizer device all through the days and nights; the woman therapist stayed at the hospital around the clock because she lived 25 miles away. No matter how I felt, I loved hearing her describe the woods and fields around her trailer home, how she heard the birdcalls break into the silence.

Nurses gave me injections every few hours, some new life-saving therapy just approved from Canadian experiments. Of course, I had oxygen tubes and I.V.'s.

I had so wanted to die I told my closest Aide friend when he came to visit me in intensive care that I was smiling. "I'm not smiling!" he replied.

I wanted to apologize to my beloved roommate, Edith, for keeping her awake that wild night. She sent a nature photo and note to me but had new troubles of her own. Her naturopath daughter ordered a strictly darkened, private room for Edith, so when I was sent back to the home, I could not even wheel in to see her. I put a sign on our door (now no longer mine, too) "motor-mouth is gone from this room".

I do recall saying something quite loudly and foolishly as I passed physical therapy and saw the Director. Something about my being back again! Too bad for her I was not discharged. Silly. In-jokes. My P.T. had to resume with the beginning exercises.

However, it was to the Aide, Ryan, I revealed my inner thoughts. Ryan, the big young tribal man who himself was on a slippery slope. He had left the reservation and tried to finish secondary school but a chronic blood problem made him miss months of classes, so he dropped out. Now, he worked two jobs, shared living quarters with acquaintances who later stole music equipment he'd extravagantly bought. One leech was still with him, wanting to party while he tried to study for his G.E.D. and train in hospital work. Ryan wanted to continue as a CNA while he would study to be a registered nurse. Oh, what a good nurse he could be, and strong, big males are in short supply.[8]

Ryan had depth. Ryan had patience. He somehow took time for talk—as healing as his ancestors who must have been medicine men and women. So I asked him if God was giving me retribution for not being understanding in the thirteen years my mother lived in my home. I even had been angry with God, said he must have gone to Acapulco on vacation, when he kept her lingering, limp, unable to speak, and needing a Hoyer lift[9]. How her eyes had raged!

Ryan listened, and then quietly said, "I've observed the elders choose when to die".

"But she'd always dreaded becoming bedridden!"

––––––––––––––––––––

[8] True for Bert and 4 a.m. whirlpool baths

[9] Sling like Edwina's.

"I've observed," he went on, "some elders refuse to die. They hang on, waiting…"

"For some joy they had not had?"

"Perhaps. Or just not wanting to be quitters."

"Or to say goodbye?" Long ago, my co-worker told how her gravely ill mother, who lived in a distant town, waited for her to arrive and then peacefully died.

Ryan said he'd seen that occur in the Home, "Some here have no one; they die from boredom or emptiness. Some hold off for many reasons."

"But I should have been kinder to her."

"Don't keep blaming yourself. Making peace with an elder takes many forms. When she went, she must have felt peace was made."

Bless that young Native American, wherever he is. I asked about Ryan at the restaurant where he worked his second job. He was gone. Moved away somewhere.

Chapter VIII

Summing Up

My personal experiences in the skilled nursing facility were tempered by factors not possible for a long-term patient. I had not given up my world and I was heading back to mobility, normalcy -- hopefully. The apathy nursing home clients feel is understandable but it is destructive. Except for the gravely ill, bedridden patient, a nursing home resident can choose to interact with others and engage in available stimulation or succumb to tempting apathy. The hours between daily procedures: getting up and dressed; hours between meals and then evening hygiene can easily slip away. Some clients just sit, unmotivated, and eventually live up to the cliché: "Use it or lose it."

Dr. Roger Walsh, psychiatrist at the University of California Medical School, and Dr. Marian Diamond, his colleague, have conducted studies on nerve cells. Their conclusions disprove the old adage that brain function involving nerve cells diminishes. "Stimulated nerve cells of the brain can grow!"

In their studies directly applied to the aging brain, Dr. Walsh and Dr. Diamond insist, "We are doing older people a disservice by laying our negative expectations on them." This report was printed in the

Dallas Morning News, Dallas, Texas newspaper about 1990.

I observed the choices a human spirit can make, and you will meet the individuals in Part II of my experiences *FROM THE INSIDE* who remained vibrant even though they spent years in an institutional existence.

One lady of 94 said it best in valentines she made for her grandchildren, complete with a smiling photo of herself in the whirlpool bath:

> I hope your day is happy.
> I am making mine that way.
> For the despondent,
> every day brings trouble.
> Have a happy heart!
> Echo of Auntie Mame
> There is a feast if you look for it,
> so "don't go hungry."

You'll meet the Lady in Red who challenged a guest speaker at our facility:

"Don't sell us short. Everyone has to get old and we learn to cope." And to help others as this 96 year-old, true Lady did for her fellow residents. I watched what I missed as a visitor: bonding between people enclosed together which can wipe away ugliness of disabilities; patients and staff know the real persons shining through frailty. To many demented clients reality is their past, considered better than now.

J. Friedman of *Earth's Elders Foundation* observed "those who have outlived everything but their memories". I believe many are not 'out to lunch' and you will meet Altha Mae in the next section of *FROM THE INSIDE.*

I met many men and women, fellow inmates of my nursing home, by wheeling beside them or, when appropriate, into their rooms. They were invigorated as we talked and re-lived their lives. Sharing stories was easier because I was a patient, too. I elicited some smiles from the sign taped on the back of my wheelchair, STUDENT DRIVER. Fragile Claire, described earlier, saw me struggling to wheel myself out sliding glass doors open to a patio. She surprised herself by vigorously pulling my chair from outside. We were all in this existence together.

Modern, well-run nursing homes publicize patients' rights. In some, patients elect a Council who presents their complaints to the administration. I have described many wise activities, and I did see much gentleness for bedridden patients. You'll meet Edwina.

A patient shaky from traumas leads to the need for a skilled nursing facility. The client may have had surgery or broken bones, so undergoes rehabilitation in a program of Physical Therapy (P.T.). Then there are goals for self-help for daily tasks, especially when a patient has become weak, debilitated but is considered potentially able to return to normal living at home. Such tasks are practiced under the direction of Occupational Therapy (O.T.). Stroke victims can be in rehab, as can accident victims and people with chronic illnesses that have taken a bad turn—diabetes, lung problems, some cancers in remission or cleared, and the client has to gain strength and mobility. Rehab is a positive reason to be in a nursing home. My experience was such, but I circulated among people who were permanent patients for reasons of medical necessity, no hope of recovery, or—more often—because there was no one to take care of them. I did not probe, therefore, did not know, the private medical problems of the Lady in Red nor of the musically gifted man and wife, nor of the Cowboy's various rough-tough roommates. Their vibrancy was in belligerence.

Living on is described in text and photographs in Jerry Fieldman's first book, *Earth's Elders*, many of whom he interviewed in nursing homes. Mr. Friedman overcame his stereotypic view of passive folk lined up in wheelchairs, one who curtly waved his photographer away. The man did not want to speak, quite the opposite of a 100-year-old gentleman who joyfully left his card game to talk about baseball. He kept up with his favorite team, could list years of their scores. He agreed with Mr. Friedman that one must "use it or lose it", and that the word 'worry' comes from an ancient root word 'to choke,' and how we all must "maintain positivism at any age."

Dr. Zorba Pastor wrote *Longevity Code* along with Susan Meltsner of New York Three Rivers Press, in 2001. The book emphasizes: "A negative or self-blaming attitude can end lives prematurely. Our thoughts are powerful. They can lift some depression, can stabilize blood pressure, and even bring cholesterol levels down."

I want you to meet individuals I came to know and love, clients in my nursing home who shared their life stories. I do not use their real names.

Recording memories is being valued by Story Corps[10], largest oral history project in America. Brainchild of Dave Ismay and published by Penguin Press, the book *Listening is an Act of Love* proves we all have "significant personal relevancy," and we feel "thrilled someone cares to listen." Jerry Friedman continued to do so in his second study, *Talks with Elders Worldwide*, again many of whom were in nursing homes.

We will go on with my observations, my experiences *FROM THE INSIDE.* I introduced myself to:

> "the most important aspect of our existence -- people by not shutting out the staggering richness of our living world."

These words are from Robert P. Harrison of Stanford University in his *Gardens, an Essay on the Human Condition*, University of Chicago Press, 2008.

Picture a large, really large, mustard-colored cowboy hat. I wheeled up to the man under it and exclaimed, "What a great hat!"

Harold drawled, "You betcha! Given to me by a movie star. He saw me win a horse race."

Approaching Altha Mae, a tidy little lady, moving on in deliberate steps, holding her Bible against her side I said, "Your hair is beautiful."

---

[10] http://storycorps.org/record-your-story/what-to-expect/

The Cowboy bumped my wheelchair with his extended leg in its cast. He delighted in shocking me.

On to Norma, the bitter, wry lady with her California clothes. I wheeled into her room and exclaimed, "All the Hollywood photos!"

"They're of my grandson. See, there he is with John Wayne."

In Edwina's room, I looked up at the ceiling above her bed. Edwina, tall, large, with luminous brown eyes, had to lie flat. Therefore, dozens of kitten pictures were pasted on her ceiling. In the ten years I knew Edwina, her bulletin board held only a few photos of herself with a trio of laughing friends; Edwina gazing at a baby on a bed; and several of an overly made-up blonde-haired woman, her daughter whom I never met.

Honey, the candy lady, a patient in a different rest home was bright little woman. She was Director of Purchasing, Sales, Marketing and Accounting for her facility's candy concession. When I met Honey I learned how she lived up to her name and how she operated from her wheelchair. She talked with patients to decide what candy would sell. Having always been a whiz at math, she had kept books for her salesman husband. Honey managed the money from candy sales and she made out order slips for the wholesale candy supplier. She not only was a merry little lady, but an example of psychologists' dictum not to give in to apathy.

Sailing through the halls of my nursing home was the Lady in Red. How coy could one get, I foolishly thought: the walker on wheels and the grinning lady in a different outfit everyday. Always in red along with her bright rouge, she would be waving a red stuffed animal. How wrong was my reaction!

This lady was 96. I visited her when I finally caught up as she flew down the hall, and I came to know a powerhouse, a skilled craftsman. Her room was beautiful. The tidy shelves were filled with handmade dolls and soft animals. Over tables and her bed were red crocheted coverlets and shawls, which along with the dolls and animals she gave away. "Cheers people up, especially the red."

She didn't have to explain the wearing of the red, the rouge; how dense I had been. How often we sneer, stop to pray and then stand in awe and respect. I looked forward to the Lady in Red's companionship. I sat with her at a lecture on aging. The speaker asked for people's reactions. The Lady in Red stood up and projected to the farthest corners of the Day Room, as she had done weeks before, "Don't play us down! Old is wise. Old is the end of push, of worry, and is the time to smile. To brighten up where you are!"

When some listeners objected and said they were all "down" in this home, the Lady retorted, "No, here we're learning the ability to cope! And we all MUST learn to cope. We're all going to be old and will need care!"

June A. W. Severance

PART II

Life Stories of Beloveds

June A. W. Severance

Fred B.

There was great variety among the patients, some new, some long-time residents of the Home. One who could not speak was a pitiful little lady who sat, always by herself, twisting in her wheelchair. We waved. She pointed to Wanda as she passed. Wanda had a thin, musical voice, but did not converse, just calling, calling as she pushed her walker with small steps, often dangerously uncertain, but her presence was as constant in the Day Room as the dignified gentleman who moved restlessly sometimes encountering the Cowboy, a meeting that often meant a blow-up. This gentleman listened to daily newspaper reading and current event talks by staff members. He liked the music programs and the Saturday matinee movies, but – and I respected this – said, "I prefer not to chat." He did enjoy the finches flitting in and out of their nests built within glass cases in the Day Room.

I wheeled over to meet a tall woman who had just settled herself.

"Are you from the West?" I guessed right.

"Yes, I always ranched from childhood, but here I am in a Nursing Home. All I can think of are the days I rode my horse all over the hills – all day, just me and the horse and my dog following along, all over the hills."

"I share such memories and longings."

Fred had regrets and longings, too, but wit and gracious sweetness came with his words: "I climbed every mountain out where I used to live. Every peak in the Pioneers and up in the other ranges, too."

"Now," He smiled, not piteously, just realistically when he added, "Now I can't even walk."

However, he was famous in art galleries, big cities and small, as well as restaurants, schools, and in every wing of the facility. Fred's photographs were shown in all those places.

"Two thousand negatives I have -- scenes of the rural West, of animals, of the Dakota's first Territorial Capitol."

The photos were an eternal tribute in their professional clarity and composition. Fred never seemed "frail or elderly" which he was, but rather the epitome of a Gentleman, the perfect white hair and trimmed beard, the clean shirt and white sweater-jacket. He could have been your family dentist or beloved uncle. Actually, Fred had been a city businessman and an outdoorsman. He said, "It started from boyhood when my Oregon mother would run with us to the creek where the best berries grew."

Once an intrepid mountaineer, now he became the smiling listener and conversationalist. Even when he was short of breath he told how he'd gone up in small planes. That led us into talking about my husband's World War II air adventures. The only gently cross words I ever heard Fred say were after another chiding I gave him about not eating his meals.

"No," he retorted, pushing the plate away. "I don't like the menu!"

Fred and I would linger after dinner; we'd smile over our likes and dislikes -- especially our love of mountains. Finally, Mr. B. would give in and resignedly say, "I'd better roll back to my room. Early to bed."

I agreed with Fred, as we prepared to roll, although some evenings I wanted to see the sky, even catch a sunset from a window in the door of a certain wing, that is, if someone could help me there.

Of the three night shift Aides named Mary, yes, three blessed Mary's one was particularly kind. She remembered I liked two overnight-gowns. This Mary hurried about, even offered back rubs and that extra, assisted bathroom trip. Charts were on bathroom doors for Aides to record urinary output. Mary and I wondered if there was a winner of the most output in all of USA.

June A. W. Severance

Bert

Not all residents in homes are elderly, there are people like Bert. He was the gentleman I gave my desserts to until I learned he should not eat sweets.

"Never thought I'd be in here," Bert said. "I was one of the people who started this place; three of us ranchers, some local merchants and a doctor. We decided this part of our state was lacking a rehab place to heal and a place for elderly folks so if they needed permanent care their families wouldn't be too far away."

"Must have been hard work raising the money."

I could see Bert thinking "...pretty obvious. Lot of flack when we sold out. The facility has been here over thirty years."

"But this place looks new!"

"The nursing home chain redecorated when they took over. Made government mandated changes. Set up the Physical Therapy unit – tops in the state – and you know how those O.T. people even check on patients' homes."

I laughed at the idea of Occupational Therapy but replied, "People who leave here really know what they can and can't do back home."

I was tempted to tease Bert about missing so many P.T. sessions, but I stopped when he started to defend himself.

"This 'rest' facility is no place for rest. I just get through breakfast, meet up with my son to run over the day's ranch decisions and then lie down. I'm supposed to be healing but some bimbo comes in and chortles, 'I have to take your vitals.'"

"Oh, Bert, I know. I tell them they're welcome to my vitals. Take 'em away!"

Bert laughed, "And do you know what time the Aides take me for a bath?"

"No when?"

"Four in the morning. Worse than the Army."

"More male Aides on night shift."

"And with my girth I need them. Really, it's no problem. For that whirlpool, I'll go anytime."

"Yes, I never knew patients had to be up early and dressed. I guess it's good discipline and stimulation."

"Not for me after so much lost sleep. Aides answering lights all night. Roommate putting on call light so we both wake up." Bert yawned just talking about it.

"Do you get a jolt from that tall Aide?"

"The one with the 'Ready, get up' at 6:30? If I didn't let her help me up, she'd make the bed with me in it."

"Pity her family with a dynamo like that!"

Now Bert was serious. "I knew them, her former family. She's all alone now."

We both agreed that one did not want to bother busy Aides by delaying getting ready for breakfast.

He also knew the new lovely woman we both went to sit with, Margaret. She and my roommate were old friends and that is how I learned how Margaret was hurt in a car crash driving alone. How she lost her son a year ago.

Margaret only told of the lucky side. "The police officer knew how to extricate me from the windshield, so gently. I knew him from the time my sisters and I lived in town going to high school. He herded for us on the family ranch. He knows broken bones, like broken necks."

We called Margaret our Egyptian Princess. Curved metal rods rested on shoulder cushions; they supported a metal circle actually riveted to her head. We ached for her, but she never whined; in fact, Margaret laughed how her nephews decided they'd bring colored lights to rig up on the metal circle so she could be Santa Lucia.

"How do you sleep?"

She paused, "Well, I do sleep some. But I feel for the poor lady in my room."

"Is she the one who calls hel-p, hel-p over and over?" I had wondered which room. I had told the Aide not to mind my call light but go to that pitiful voice. He said he'd been there eight times in the hour that night and every night.

Margaret also knew Georgia, age 101, who had gone to school with Margaret's mother We all talked so eagerly about history that Georgia sat up like a Dowager Queen even when family members arrived and cooed over her. Margaret and I winced, as they talked about Georgia in the third person. "She's been sleeping so much…doesn't know anyone."

One look at Georgia's sharp eyes and the firm mouth and we knew she knew that she did exist, just as much as she wished her family recognized she was really there, maybe only listening, but truly there.

Our Margaret was more pink–cheeked every day as we worked side-by-side in Physical Therapy. One morning a fluttery Assistant Activities Director approached us about taking Communion. Yes! We went to Margaret's room and held hands as we prayed first. The Director hurried in, waited a bit uncomfortably, she did have others to serve, as Margaret and I finished the Our Father and received the Host. A special moment – Margaret-of-the-crown, her quiet calm, the flowers on her bureau -- an Easter moment and for Margaret her healing was her Resurrection.

Margaret and I discussed the thoughtlessness of speaking third person in the presence of the patient. I related a story of a very dignified client who was wheeled to the Beauty Salon of another Nursing Home where I was. The beautician was working on a client and said quite loudly, "Oh, put her in the empty room over there."

The wheelchair occupant sat up, obviously very offended. She was ready to cry as she was pushed aside like a stray package.

Both the beautician from the outside and the Aide should have been corrected about their lack of sensitivity. The other insensitive talk was when Aides and others come in and say, "Let's take our medicine. We need to get up and bathe."

Several times I answered, "Okay, you take our pills this morning."

June A. W. Severance

Madeline

I was not too critical of the Assistant Activities' Director; she meant well and was so proud to be taking the Priest around the facility, telling us all how his brother was a Bishop. She worried about schedules and would bring Father to see me "if there was time." There was and he was candid and deep, a great rock-Petra, St. Peter.

The Assistant Director introduced me to her tiny mother of ninety-six years. I had seen this dear little patient walking carefully to her assigned place in the main dining room.

I said, "Such bright dark eyes."

"Oh," she said, "we all are dark, all French, down from Canada."

Madeline told me of their small place. She said, "My father kept animals and gardens and crops. There were nineteen of us."

"Nineteen children – all at home?"

"Yes we had so much laughter. We didn't have things – too many of us – but such a happy time all of us. Then Sundays when aunts and uncles and cousins came!"

"Did you have to rent a Parish hall?"

Madeline laughed and told me I must have been a town girl. "We just put boards on saw horses and ate. Everybody brought food. We danced. Played the old French tunes. Oh, we had a happy life!"

I could hear lines of poetry in the rhythm of her voice:

"A flash of wings
Outside a kitchen door!
Life's colored moments,
A patchwork quilt
Warming us as we dream."

The last time Madeline and I talked, the Assistant Director hurried over. She bent over her tiny, dark-haired mother and sadly said, "Everything about the past. She says nothing about today."

Madeline and I looked at each other, a deep look.

Let's Call Her Helen

Her family chose this certain Nursing Home because a particular longtime friend was there. In addition, the Home was near enough so family could drop in easily. The former neighbor was delighted Helen was "settling in nicely." Very soon, however, she ceased to associate with Helen, saying, "She makes me nervous. Holding a conversation is wearing on me."

She had come to realize Helen's limitations, so holding a conversation was "wearing on me." However, the longtime friend did hurry in to Helen's room when the family visited. She pretended concern and always inquired about "your dear mother, Helen. She does have good color in her cheeks…" and so on, always referring to Helen in the third person within Helen's hearing[11].

Helen was discouraged. When wheeled into the general dining room, she was embarrassed thinking everyone was staring at her. At first, doubtless because she was "the new kid on the block." A few times, she

---

[11] This is a dastardly habit people slip into when visiting.

was moved to the area for the incapacitated like Edwina. Helen wept, "Too sad. I'm giving up!"

The staff decided upon a buddy system, pairing Helen with a cheery patient who also had difficulty speaking. This resident always stopped to shake hands with everyone. The Speech Pathologist designed a program for the two ladies, especially hoping Helen would feel useful, having something we all need, purpose to get up in the morning. Would Helen help the older lady?

"No, I'm moving on. I'm no good."

"Where, Helen?"

"Where ever someone can find a place for me."

All I heard later was that Helen's depression overwhelmed her. She passed away. Some family members used the word 'senile' having given up on Helen, sure she could not learn, but facts from the National Mental Health Association asserts that Crystalline Intelligence (problem solving intelligence) actually increases with age. The vicious cycle of depression can lead to loss of learning ability.

Could Helen's discouragement, loss of energy and motivation have been diagnosed earlier and treated?

Seraphim and Cherubim

The Seraphim are Registered Nurses and Licensed Practical Nurses. The Cherubim are Certified Nurses Aides. These angels may not often be seen by visitors -- outsiders who judge nursing homes by the glimpses of bedridden patients lying on their sides or flat on their backs. Above their beds are instructions for the CNAs, whom I will refer to simply as Aides. I do not minimize their rigorous training and the test they must pass to do the direct handling of patients. Signs remind these Aides to move clients every two hours to prevent bedsores.

They wipe dry mouths with moist, flavored swabs and administer lotions on frail skin. They give bed baths and clean feces and bedpans. There is much lifting involved and infinite patience! These Certified Nurses Aides are not high on the pay scale, so there is much turnover. They do basic tasks, such as feed toothless mouths patiently even when the Aide has to help others finish their meals on schedule.

Then night shift Aides must settle in ten to a dozen or more patients and answer all-night calls, "Nurse---hel—p me." Many bedridden clients do not realize the Aide has just responded to the call light over the door and they call again, "Hel—p me!"

Without high praise and adequate recompense, Aide jobs often are undertaken until better jobs come along. I want to shout that the geriatric medical field increasingly needs more workers. An immense burden is carried by the Aides and Nurses full R.N.'s, and L.P.N.'s.

Let us begin with the dayshift. Bedridden patients need, as I said, complete cleansing and then feeding. Patients who wash and dress themselves still have to be helped out of bed into wheelchairs or to walkers and taken or guided by elbows to wash sinks with warning not to pull on nor lean on the sink while washing. It can be tugged off the wall.

The Physical Therapists do a fine job of strengthening their clients!

After each meal, Aides fill out a chart with squares indicating how much food each patient ate. In dealing with helpless clients, an Aide has to record the fluid and/or solid wastes at the time the bedpan is emptied. There are lists on bathroom doors. One Aide and I wondered if these records were filed in Washington, D.C. with the Department of Health. For all patients the VITALS (love that word) must be taken: blood pressure, pulse, temperature and breath rate.

One afternoon when I had just dozed off after the above VITALS were taken an Aide returned to my bedside. Then a full R.N. arrived. I was carefully quizzed. Was I hurting or troubled; the extremely high B/P reading suggested I was agitated. I deeply pondered. Oh! I realized the powerful love story video I had just seen in the day room had stirred me.

(I wondered if I had to tell my fantasies.) Truly, I was touched by the extra time and concern of the Aide and the Nurse.

Night shift Aides have to hustle, beginning with bedtime needs, toileting, helping with fresh hospital gowns. One Aide had her own worries. Her husband left taking their young son. Yet, she never let me feel she was in a hurry. She would offer to rub my back with lotion. She noticed the curve in my spine from an old accident when transverse bones were broken. (I always joked that a horse decided to sit down on me. Actually, a nasty mare reared and threw herself over; I still feel the crunch.) Mary always brought me two night garments so I could tie one in the back and wear the other as a wraparound to the front. Bless her. (I hope she found her little boy!) We would laugh that a patient loses all modesty in a home. Tie-in-the-back gowns should be x-rated.

Then there was the tall night Aide who worked as a short-order cook by day, and was a rod and a staff to patients like me for midnight bathroom help.

He'd step away "to give some privacy," but he cautioned me not to totter on my own to get back to the bed. His kind ways made waiting for him, as he dashed to other rooms, tolerable. Maybe I was learning patience. Nights were haunting. Silence, then med-time clatter of pill carts and, as if we patients were unconscious, loud orders, the VITALS and chitchat among the workers. In addition, lights are turned on and off.

There were errors, too. One day, I was parked in a hallway after an Aide had wheeled me from a meeting. As she locked the brakes of the chair she asked, "Are you all right here?"

Thinking she wondered if I felt secure in the chair I answered, "Yes, fine."

The Aide disappeared. I did not know where I was because the meeting had been in a part of the Home used for business matters, conference rooms instead of patients' rooms. I mused about the meeting I had just attended and my chance to voice my opinions of the facility. The germ of my writing about life *FROM THE INSIDE* began there. I could tell about the dietician's whoops of delight when I praised the food. But time passed.....and passed. I stared at a painting and its handsome frame; I began to feel I was attached to the wall just as the picture was.

I knew the rule that a patient was not to wheel away without an Aide's help or approval. Perhaps no one knew where I was. Then came the dire need for a bathroom and I was in tears. Yes, I had become vulnerable, knew firsthand how helpless a disabled person can be, how serious an Aide's mistake can be.

Another time, I was shaken figuratively by an Aide. It occurred the first time I walked by myself. The walker was put aside. I was to try walking while grasping the hall railing. I shuffled along. On subsequent strolls, I learned the staff called me the walking mummy because the elastic wraps around my legs unraveled. Only one excellent Aide successfully bound them.

That day of my first walk, I continued all the way to the Day Room. I was amazed. I just glimpsed the glass case where lovely, live Finches darted in and out of their small nests. Then I had to stagger to a chair. I was in a cold sweat. I asked an Aide for water. (I could hear my favorite Sons of the Pioneers singing, "cool, clear wa—ter!")

"I'll have to check at the Nurses' Station," the Aide replied.

"For water?"

"I have to see if there are orders for you."

"For water?" I gasped, not knowing then as I did later that some patients (like Edwina) can aspirate on water. The Aide was being cautious, but that day I only knew the room was getting fuzzy as I leaned back in the chair.

One blow-up led to my complaining about an Aide. A new young woman came on night duty and answered my light, "What do you want?"

When I told her about a wedge I needed from the closet shelf, she balked, did not know what it was nor wanted to reach for it.

"It's a foam support, in sort of a slant. Keeps me from lying flat," I explained.

"I don't want to get it!"

We blew up at each other. She did get the wedge and stormed out of the room.

My friend, the ex-Army medic, reported her but also said she shouldn't be working at the home; she'd been in jail in Canada. Time passed, the young woman softened. Perhaps she had leftover anger and problems. Everyone needs a second chance, and I heard she had been welcomed back to America by her family.

Soon she was telling me about her dogs, how she'd been given one and then bought its sister. Beautiful collies. Oh, I related to that! Somehow, I began to tell her about a nature CD of original piano music with sounds of wind and rain and rushing streams. A friend had composed this, "Sounds of Georgia."

The blonde Aide, I called "S" was excited. She said she loved music and asked if she could borrow the CD. I gave it to "S", although I was warned I would never get it back, but I did and from a beaming "S". We were friends and better people, both of us, having performed a rare change from resentment to warmth and true forgiveness.

More than a year later, I encountered "S" at a County Fair. She was leading her two beautiful collies. We hurried toward each other. "I remember you from the home!" "S" called out. "You were so nice to me."

"S" told me she had taped the music of my CD and still listened to it because it brought her such peace. We hugged and went our separate ways.

Later, I saw her picture in the obituaries of a city newspaper. She had died, no cause listed, at age 41.

To some Aides, the non- or vaguely responsive patients were "out to lunch". But you'll meet Altha, who was full of deep thoughts, very much present. Day by day, some Aides can become perfunctory, tired of constant repetition as they repeatedly swish toothbrushes in saliva-drooling mouths; lemon mouth swabs slip out or spit out. Aides are hurried and plop plates of food on the restraining wooden trays across the arms of chairs rolled out in the hall, as in my father's experience.

I chuckled over the cheery, "Are WE all set? Let's eat OUR food, ok?"

Constant OK's. What if clients said, "No!" How are "WE going to wash OUR faces" or gobble "OUR food" all jolly together?

However, my friend Fay was a compassionate Aide. As a teenager she had run away with a circus. Still young when I knew her, Fay was supporting her mother and her little girl. One midday Fay was alarmed when as always and of her own choice she came to see if I needed anything special.

I had used my grabber to pull the drapes on the circular track bolted to the ceiling above my bed. The cloth swung like a theater curtain, and I was in a cozy cave. I had also pulled the thin bedspread and pillow over my head. Only when a friend recently described her father having done the same in his nursing home bed, did I realize how my cave-urge looked. She and her mother thought her dad was dead.

Fay was alarmed! She pulled a part of the privacy drapes aside and she was almost in tears, "What's wrong? Are you...?"

"No, dear, I'm just in a lazy mood." I smiled, and I told Fay I sometimes needed to retreat into a selfish cocoon. No! I did not intend any self-destruction, and I liked the loving people in the Home. Sometimes one just cannot muster up response. Fay understood. Yes, a snug bed, a table with one's few needs, and a curtain drawn around one's space is all one wants. At certain moments, that is.

In addition, Fay and I visited each other long after I was discharged. She had done so much for me that my joy equaled hers when she married a good man and, I hope, is living somewhere "happily ever after."

At another nursing home, I met the Director of Nursing. She was mingling with the Aides who joked and smiled with patients. I was impressed with the atmosphere and with the Director's compassion as she, too, bent over the disabled people, wiping the mouth of one whose spoonful of food had not quite reached its destination.

"Working here is very different from my years in an acute care hospital. There we had to tell patients and their families the options for medical decisions. We would be pinned to the wall if we did otherwise!" The Director, Ruth, gestured. "Here we communicate in many ways with the patient. We try, if he or she can understand, but we must decide."

"And the families?" I asked.

"Often, they are almost as afraid as the patients. Most do not know what care is needed; just leave it up to us. Or there is no one."

Ruth watched as two Aides used a machine lift to get Nita, my 90-year-old friend, from recliner to wheelchair. Frustrated because she had always stood on her own two feet, been a successful career woman, my friend swore fiercely at the Aides as they took the oxygen container to the chair and gently removed Nita's nose tubes. They knew my friend was not furious with them but dismayed over what age and strokes, life itself, had done to her.

When I praised the Aides for their calm and kindness, they said, "We like helping people."

This phrase was echoed by a muscular CNA, 6'7", who told me he had been a Special Education teacher in Santa Monica for years, but wearied of the crowds.

"So I came here. It's peaceful. I'm enjoying life and still helping." He lifted my friend, making sure she had an elastic band buckled firmly around her waist. He could hold it if she slipped down. Her hands were grasping his strong arms, and I even saw her flirtatious smile when Chuck eased her into the car and surrounded her with pillows. We were going for a scenic drive.

Chuck waved. Yes, helping people. Thank Heaven for the Seraphim and Cherubim. I could go on and on – the bright ever willing Connie who worked on toenails or cheered us up with her everlasting wit. Calm Jane made P.T. a joy and a success. Night Aides who brought prayer sheets from church, so quietly blessing me. Then one night a very young, and very smart Aide stayed helping me to breathe deeply to overcome panic during a siege of atrial fibrillation[12].

Quietly Tammie said, "My mother is a nurse."

There was pride in that statement and now Tammie is in nursing school, specializing in Geriatrics[13].

------

[12] A-Fib feels like a rock band percussion frenzy where your heart should be.

[13] I saw how she beguiled the frailest elderly.

June A. W. Severance

Altha Mae

Now to a special little lady, whom some Aides said was non-responsive, "out-to-lunch" in their words. In fact, they believed the patient's family visited less often because she really did not know them. We will use the name Altha Mae.

I first met her as she retrieved her Bible from the top of the piano. She had just finished playing for patients in the Nursing Home. She tucked the Bible in the crook of her arm against the waistband of her blue skirt, made sure her spanking white blouse was tucked in. We had spoken a few words when she politely excused herself. "Because I need to get to my work now."

I watched the heavy black oxfords move sturdily out of the Day Room and down the hall to her room where her name was on a pretty sign. "Altha Mae" – letters surrounded by small flowers. She explained a few days later, when I had wheeled into her room making sure she was finished with her work. Every day she marked prophecies in the Old Testament that were fulfilled in the New. I told Altha Mae how my father knew another lady who did that.

"Where is she?" Altha Mae asked.

"Far away in Iowa."

I remarked about the embroidery on her white blouse. Over the years, I noticed she always wore a white blouse.

"My daughter and I came across it 'way down in a pile of things packed to store at her house. That's her portrait."

She pointed to a fine photo that looked like a younger Altha Mae. In the years Altha Mae and I were friends, I never encountered her daughter at the Nursing home.

It is so difficult to convey the essence of the tidy, little patient, a permanent resident of the Home, her lovely hair remained mahogany brown in all the eight years I visited her. Worn in a bun, her hair was smoothed in place with combs. I often saw Altha Mae take each comb out and re-smooth her hair. She was immaculate. Her room was "neat as a pin." Bless the Aides for the help they must have given each day, as Altha Mae said, "Here I feel like a blessed human being."

She, like Norma, had been brought to this Nursing Home to be near the family, but the daughter believed Altha Mae didn't even know them and "there wasn't anything to talk about."

All I know is that her wisdom, her epigrams stirred me and gave me peace. The quicksilver words now that I also am in my eighties have been absorbed and have changed me.

One day Altha Mae showed me a newspaper photo and asked me to put it on her bulletin board. "This picture is my sister. She was tall and handsome."

The news story described the excellent therapy for Alzheimer victims at our Nursing Home. I studied the picture, the fine boned face, the deep expression of the eyes. Certainly, this was Altha Mae herself, but she continued, "My sister there in the photo had been a teacher."

"Did you teach, too?" I asked carefully; I had noted Altha Mae's good vocabulary.

"Oh, I just went in to help; I loved the children of all ages and my boys were in the school. We had the big ones help the little ones. Why, we could even teach the same history lessons to all at the same time!"

I was amazed as Altha Mae described the lesson plans. "But you know you go in slowly. Children live their own pace. They watch you. They'll only let you in after a while."

Her voice was drifting. I wanted her to continue. "When children get to know you?"

"As time passes, yes, and as they trust you inside," to demonstrate, Altha held her hands together against her heart, against her thin chest. When I hugged her, I felt only one set of bones, front and back. I knew then why she was in the special, assisted eating-place. I wanted to preach about eating more but I held off. She never complained of being ill, "Oh, just a bit of weakness, nothing more, and really all over now."

She had come from a place poetically called Plentyland. "It's where the Ross families first came."

"From Scotland?" Names came to me: I'd been in Wester – Ross along the Outer Minch.

"Some. Some of my family were from England. It was said they went to some dark state first."

"Perhaps Kentucky. That was called the dark and bloody ground."

"Yes! I remember that from the history books, but mama never said. There were ten of us and she died with the last baby; they were buried together in the same box, mama and the tiny baby."

Altha caught her breath and went on. "Papa had to work so hard to take care of all of us and everything on the ranch. We had a garden. Had to break ice even in spring and carry water from along ways away. But Plentyland was happy. I loved the animals! He had a special breed, and, of course, the cattle. In summer, they'd go up on the bench where there were acres and acres of wild grasses, the old Indian bunch grasses. The most nutritious there are.
My brothers always hurried to get the chores done so they could get to riding. The boys would simply give their calls from the fence rail and even the wildest-seeming horses would come running, holding their heads up proud, manes flying. For days, the boys would be riding them to get to the cows and back – summer and fall. Yes, we had big crops, too. Some winters we had to move into town so the boys could go to high school.

Again, the few pictures on the bulletin board brought the present in line with the past. Altha Mae's own boys had ranched. There she was, tiny between two husky men. "Yes, my boys and their big-car vehicle. They have a trucking business. I call them boys still because they know they can always come to us at the ranch and we'll always help them."

Again, Altha put her hands to her heart, pressing them to go with her words, "What's deep inside."

There was a photo of a small dog, which she said was the king, "If anything wrong was ever done to him even when he wails over his bath, the roof would fall in at the ranch." In the snapshot, Altha's daughter was seated near the dog and she was holding one of the children; another child was at the fireplace of what seemed a suburban-type home. Altha Mae did not acknowledge any more about the picture.

One time when Altha Mae finished playing the piano, people asked her to play her accordion, too. She did. Then she abruptly left the Day Room for "her work." She went in an almost sliding movement, her feet becoming tender. She instructed me on cleaning suede shoes like hers. It was a very precise method. As I saw her in the hall, I waved and her eyes would light up.

"Altha Mae. I was looking for you."

"And I for you. I just passed the hall where you always used to be and there was a vacant place." She did not know I'd been discharged a long while ago but had been coming to the facility to see my friends and to see her.

"I'll always find you. You're my friend."

"That is the best word anyone can say or hear."

We agreed on how different sorts of people should get to know one another, "and then co-operate." As she and I could not "contradict one another; we'd just be contradicting ourselves." How tender and wise!

A strange visit occurred one day. I sat with Altha Mae at the Home's musical show. She perched at the edge of her chair, puzzled. "Nothing seems right. If I could just get to my house. I need to get in home but I don't have the key."

Her eyes were alert, startled. The dark eyes like those of a wonderful horse about to bolt. "I've felt restless the past two days, Altha Mae. Ominous." I confessed.

"What do you think? As if something wrong is about to happen."

Then we both agreed as we went back to her room. "Nothing did. Everything's all right."

"I know," she said softly, "just different."

"Altha Mae, home is around us." I cupped my hands, circled my arms. "As if God is around us and we're home."

She agreed. Her face softened and her hands came up in her customary way against her heart and then she patted the ruffle on her starched, white blouse. She talked of coming to a bigger town far from Plentyland to stay with some people who had small children.

"I helped them with the little ones. I had work."

I said, "I did that too. Good preparation for taking care of our grandchildren, like my younger one. He wants to read, loves words but they think he's not talking. They worry he'll be behind."

"Oh, sometimes that happens to children in the school. The others race ahead and want to say it all."

"Even his brother..."

"My boys at the ranch, the big one takes over." She finished my blurted sentences; Altha was herself again.

Weeks later, I asked if she was eating well and she proudly told me she was not in the assisted (feeding) dining room. But her right hand had bones and veins so prominent and red-blue splotches. (I remembered my mother's hands in the years at our home as she progressed into her nineties and on to one hundred one years old.) I said to Altha, "Broken blood vessels?"

"Bet you a nickel you're right! I'm moving it now. It was stiff; I was afraid I'd hurt it."

"Altha, I think the circulation is better this minute. You did it!" She was flexing the hand.

"I'm feeling braver! It helps to have someone say, 'you can.'" She held my hand.

I had not said those exact words but she felt them. "You have spunk, Altha Mae."

"THANK YOU." Altha had a way of stopping when we reached a high point. The concluding point. "So nice to visit. I'll look for you again."

And the next time Altha Mae ended our talk by saying, "I have to get the dinner on. I haven't even started the potatoes! The menfolk like their mashed potatoes and roast at noontime."

At a still later visit, I could see the brown eyes fading as Altha sat on the side of her bed. I asked, "Would you like to lie back on the pillow?"

"Yes, that would be nice."

I put my arm across her shoulders, bones so sharp, so frail. I made sure that the pillow was under her head. Altha Mae smoothed her cotton skirt, put her skippered feet tight together; her feet were too swollen and painful for the sturdy shoes. I can still see the toes pointed up.

"The coverlet?" I reached for the afghan so neatly folded at the end of her bed.

"Yes nice. I made that one time," her voice fainter. "And the shawl, that would be nice..."

Her words floated in the quiet. "We will meet at Heaven's gate. I'll play the music. There we'll meet with the Lord at Heaven's gate." And then – Altha Mae stirred. "The work isn't done. I must put dinner on."

Tears caught in my throat. I had shown her my latest greeting card with blue flowers she liked. I tacked it on her bulletin board beside the usual photos. However, an almost frightened look had come into her eyes.

"They're coming for me the whole family. Some were at the other house. They'll be here any minute now!"

I brought her a glass of water. Then the brown eyes softened and, "Yes some cool water would be nice. Thank you and the Lord will bless...bless you and keep you."

She clawed at the blanket with her blue-veined hands.

When I came again two days later, I knew before I reached her doorway that Altha Mae's pretty sign and her name would be gone.

An Aide hurried over. "She died yesterday, she was ready, so peaceful."

Altha Mae of Plentyland where the bunch grass pastures were never touched by a plow but wave in the wind toward Heaven's gate.

June A. W. Severance

Edith My Roommate

Edith, who looked like Jessica Tandy, was tall even as she leaned forward in a wheelchair to deal with the pain in her spine. She acknowledged our hasty meeting; her family was escorting her into our room as I was being wheeled out for some treatment. I would get to know the two daughters I met that day, know them very well as they brought food to Edith all hours of the day and night. The Naturopath, older daughter, just in from California, concocted three vegetarian meals every 24 hours. Even after her return to the west coast, her presence was felt by phone every day.

Edith and I connected the first evening and on into the night. I knew we were kindred spirits when she said, "From my kitchen window I can see a great mountain range. When there's snow, I call it white icing. No wonder the Indians called them the 'Shining Mountains'."

Edith and I were disembodied voices from our beds across the room. She was lower because her know-it-all daughter had replaced the mattress with a narrow longhaired fur pallet. At first glimpse, I thought a gray wolf had joined us.

Though confined Edith could exercise her long legs. In fact, we planned a circus act. Edith would put her feet in the 'trapeze,' a metal triangle that hung over her pallet (used for a patient to raise herself by grabbing it with both hands.) Edith used her two feet for swinging as we both warbled the song from "My Fair Lady" about a fine night for something. The Aides thought we were hilarious and the maintenance man, summoned to our room for a midnight bathroom repair, said he would do a tap dance and be the ringmaster. Our room rang with laugher. Edith and I always resolved to go back to sleep after a night interruption, having to ring an Aide for help, but another laugh would tempt us, another topic, like sheep.

"On our smaller ranch, I finally had my sheep, beauties they were," Edith was beginning. "Well, one morning Conrad, my late husband who was a dyed-in-the-wool cowman – (I apologize for the pun where ever you are, Con) - had to move some stubborn heifers and my sheep were blocking the gate. I heard a terrific rumpus. Con was yelling at the flock and making his horse charge after them. I bundled up, whistled for my dogs and went to the fray. The dogs nipped a few heels, swung around the sheep and I led the flock out of the way, their heads nodding, meek as the lambs they'd been. Conrad stopped fuming. Could I even dare to say he looked a bit sheepish as I called out to him, 'My Dear, you drive cows but I lead sheep'."

Edith was proud of all she had learned living on the big ranches owned by Conrad's family. "Later, after he died, the neighbors looked over my pastures and the good crops my youngest daughter and I raised. We took over the small ranch and ran it alone. I'd always wanted to be a truck driver, loved running machinery. Everything but the swather. Good thing my daughter was brave about that thing."

"What's a swather?" I asked.

"Hard to explain. Cuts a wide row of alfalfa, crushes it and leaves the fodder lying in a line for the baler. Nevertheless, you sit facing the back, and then right is left as the thing pushes through the grasses... There's a sort of counter balance out ahead of the driver's seat. It's a hard one. Have I confused you enough?"

"Completely. I never even drove a tractor."

"Bet you could. Most folks thought we couldn't run the place but at harvest, the heads of wheat had a count of sixty-eight kernels. Oh, how the neighbor men gawked! Then they took to complaining about their wool weigher charging more than he was paying us. Talk, talk. Swearing, sweating but no action. I went right to the source. You know how a woman can put things nicely and still demand. In a week, I received a new check, reimbursing me five cents a pound and our fleece was 130 pounds each. Oh, my rancher friends were surprised, I'll say sheepish at the money they got back, too. Then the next howl when our alfalfa was judged the best in the whole county," Edith continued.

"All the ranches together that Con's family owned added up to thousands of acres. His father had come from Europe, a farmer boy who had dared to court the area's richest maiden, too young to marry and certainly NOT to a fellow from the impoverished hills.

He emigrated to the American West, learned the ways of the prairie and bought up land 'dirt cheap'." Edith loved puns.

"The European heiress came of age and begged to be allowed to visit an American friend from boarding school. She dared to remain in America and marry the farm boy, Con's father. They made Conrad work hard, do everything hired hands did. Yes, he learned to manage all they acquired. How to run cattle, crops and people."

Edith always described her late husband as a figurehead, a strong man, but distant.

"And you learned ranching too?" I knew Edith had married from town life.

"There was certain protocol. As the owner's wife, I was not to mingle with the help, except, of course to give directions, plan meals with the cook – oh, especially during bull sales and harvesting. We had crowds to feed." she added, "I remember Harold's Ellie, finished clearing up one meal and starting the next, working beside her husband, a line cook."

Edith went on. "Then I had enough to do as the four children came on – 4-H, sports, picnics, and Con was away." Edith added, "I was told never to go out to the corrals or the animal sheds."

"Did it seem you might be flirting or the men with you?"

She told me, the men knew their place. We could joke about impossible things even as the tedious days stretched into months, as she lay flat on her pallet.

"Oh, I could watch the new foals from the ranch yard with Con's mother and visitors. I learned a lot."

Then there was the traveling. Conrad competed in sharp shooting even in Europe. "I always had clothes ready for meetings, and, oh, conventions and big parties. I hated to shop, still do, so a clothing store owner in town knew what I could wear and she'd bring out samples when she went to fashion shows."

As I listened, I could picture Edith, tall and slim, too thin now, stylish in just the right tailored suit or dress. The storeowner I met later described Edith glowingly in an English riding habit, perfect fit, the tweed jackets, always the "way she wore the outfits – with style!" Edith herself never bragged, just enjoyed remembering as our talk would ease the painful nights until growing into dawn when we would see the big willow trees outside our window.

Edith and Con were together in Alaska where he shot a grizzly, a real prize, but she did not go on the European trips. Her mother-in-law worried about their both being gone "across the pond" and the children left at home. Edith's voice took on a special flowing tone about the hat. A top hat Con bought in Paris. "The kind that collapses. He showed me this flat thing, and then punched it up, all shiny and black. Pride of his life."

"Like Fred Astaire. You can use it in the circus act."

"I did use it. At a ball!" The room rang with the warmth of her laugh. "I dressed up as a man in tails. How I swirled around the dance floor – I loved to dance – tipping the hat!"

Edith told about the first Ball she attended, the big social event of the town's 400 "I was just in my teens. Well, I saw a red satin dress with a train swishing around, a daring dress of the roaring '20s. The whole evening stays in my memory. I was dazzled because of that red gown and the woman who wore it. Not that I was ever like her. I was always in sports. I could hardly get home and back at lunchtime to practice. In college, I shot a basket from the centerline, twice! Con never really believed I did."

"I believe you." And I do. I'll stick with anything she could tell me; Edith is always in my heart. The chatelaine; the true Lady of town and ranch; the smiling leader not driver, the realist whose bones failed her. I'm sure she is among those shining mountains she longed to see again from her kitchen window.

The Cowboy

Edith said she'd been taken to Chicago to see Buffalo Bill in the Wild West Show when she was five years old.

"Yes," my friend, Russ, said.

"That's possible as the show was in spring 1918 and Edith was at the Ball in the '20s."

"Buffalo Bill died November of 1918." Russ said.

When I asked, "What's your life's work?"

He proudly answered my question with one word, "Cowboy!"

He regarded Edith as protocol demanded; she was an owner's wife. No offense, just different roles. Russ wasn't one to palaver although we had many long talks. While at the Nursing Home together in P.T., we would exchange grins; for instance, the young woman physical therapist was teaching him to flex his useless hand, disabled from the first stroke. He would dutifully squeeze the NERF ball, and then make a toss with the silly sponge ball. Later he and I devised a firmer ball of rolled up socks and practiced in his room. The Cowboy, was determined to return to his remote cabin with its dirt floor and shutters spiked against the bears, to live alone again with his beloved dog. His blue eyes flashed Labradorite to scare the

Aides as he told about the claw marks on his cabin door. Russ had been able to go back up in the mountain cabin after the first broken hip, but the staff worried. The blue eyes had the telltale white edges around the pupils. How could Russ drive that old truck of his up those twisting hills after he closed every bar in town?

We experienced those indescribable hills, vertical with deep, gashed valleys when my husband took Russ along on my first car ride. Pointing out cabins, few and far between and other people surviving in this terrain, I think he enjoyed testing us as he gave directions to old mine sites: Iron Mask, Dutchman, Dead Hole, up and down road-less gravel "slides." He had demonstrated Mountain Man skills at Frontier Fairs all over the West even after injuries and hospital stays. "I'll take whatever is dished out."

The Cowboy did begin to walk again and his feet tapped with the music of a film about a wagon train. He was holding M.T.'s hand. I was so glad to watch his intensity, the same beaming fierceness flaring up when he leaned forward – year later – in a chair and told of hunting again and shooting at the varmint who shot his horse. "Thought it was a slow Elk!"

It was interesting how Russ took to our younger autistic grandson. "He kept his distance at first, smart kid. You never know about strangers. But when he got to talking to me, he's quite a boy!"

Their eyes flashed the same sparkling blue. "He has a personality that will keep going and going. It's like he's thinking, looking at everything."

"Yes, it takes one to know one."

One day Russ said, "The first of my ancestors came from Ireland to the state of Maine, then across into New York State. He met and married my great-grandma there. Then on across the Northern territories to Oregon. Ranched. Lost one place then made a fortune with fruit trees, all kinds, in Jacksonville."

"One son of ours was married there, just across from some of those orchards. Apricots."

"And you don't touch even a withered one or you land in jail," he continued. "My father worked for the railroad and the family moved wherever he was needed. I was born in Kentucky horse country and remember Idaho the next horse country where we lived. Dad had a good job there as a brakeman. I was bringing him some food, noontime, and I watched as he jumped from one car to another. I saw him grab a handle. He was no further away than that tree."

We were talking on the patio at the edge of the shady lawn.

Russ continued, "The freight jerked forward. I saw my father fall between the cars. They started to move and rolled over him. I was five."

Russ stopped for a moment. I could see the dark-haired little boy, how he tried not to see that man cut up there before his eyes.

"My mother told me she got $6,000.00 for the funeral." I told her later. "That wasn't much for my father's life. My mother was Cherokee."

"So that's where the high cheekbones came from," I commented. I had so many questions. "How did she raise her brood of children? Did she fold her man in her arms or was he carried off? Did the boy run home or did she run to him carrying his baby brother?"

"She raised all five of us even when money ran out. You know, you grew up in the Depression. Then World War II came. Two of my brothers were killed. One was used by the Japs for bayonet practice; I identified the body by a birthmark on what was left of him. Heard just the other day that someone sold the Spokane Ranch. Hope it wasn't to Japs. They killed my brothers and now they're buying up everything."

Russ fought in the South Pacific on Saipan, stayed in the Marines thirteen years; he was wounded in Korea. He came back west, did the things he loved and knew best, "being a cowboy." Did well.

"Had a place picked out to buy but I was hurt on the job and laid off. No insurance. But a friend called me about a job with him."

Russ left the hospital there in Ely, Nevada with all his possessions. I asked if they all fit in the bag he had beside him at the moment, having been moved from his former room because he lost his temper at his night-roaming roommate. I knew the bags: big, green plastic ones labeled PATIENTS BELONGINGS[14].

"I worked ranches. First one I went to, the head wrangler said, 'See that rawboned horse over there. If you can ride him, he's yours.' Well, I caught him, let him buck himself out a little and then I took him down to the creek near the corral. Old Indian trick. The

---

[14] See Appendix. Page 126 (I) **Personal property.**

water was pretty deep. I rode him and rode him; pushing through that water cooled off the bucking." The Labradorite eyes shone. "Besides if he did throw me, I'd land in the water instead of the hard ground. But he was worn out. So I just rode him back where everyone was watching. I got the job and later the horse, too."

We were riding in our car again. My husband knew how Russ enjoyed that.

"The ranch was the one where we just stopped and the new owner's young wife gave us the water. Over 2,000 acres in that spread and I pushed herds from there over to the far end of the state. Same family both spreads."

Earlier, Edith told how her father-in-law kept the land in the family and her sister-in-law sold the ranch she inherited. That was the one we visited and Russ pointed to the same cookhouse and the bunkhouses where he'd lived, "Everything kept up fine."

I didn't look directly at him in the back seat where he was propped up with pillows, pronged cane near his good hand and medical supplies in special containers. I knew the hidden, private devices secret bags, catheters, braces with their wraps, the ones Russ was supposed to be wearing for his swelling arm. No, I didn't look, because I was thinking of all the herding years, in the great spaces of the West and of his personal triumphant ride through Deschutes Mounatins, over the Cascades to Grants Pass, Oregon where he surprised his grandparents.

"I rode alone. Yes, my favorite horse, along with one pack animal and me. Four months."

My friend brought about another's dream. Russ told of a half-brother. "A lot younger than me. Smart. Spent a lot of time with me. Well, his high school got him some scholarship and told him he should go into Engineering, everyone was getting good jobs in that. He came to me. Told me how he hated the courses. We talked while we worked on my guns, like the antique one I told you about. The boy really knew all the parts, loved working with his hands. I started talking about not doing something everybody's doing; maybe do something that was a specialty that people might need. We heard of a gun-making repair school down in Nevada: he sailed through the courses, was hired before he had his diploma and want to the big company back East. Yes, Remington and he's their pride. They bring him a gun, any kind, any age, and he can repair it right away. Identifies rare ones. Really happy, has a house there and a family."

The Cowboy's money saved to buy a ranch of his own sent the half-brother to school. He was tidy, immaculate, his reading books lined up beside his bed, "I'll have to get out of here soon or I'll go batty. Stiffening up. Oh, yes, I go to the exercises but I used to walk two, three miles a day with the dogs. Most all I ate was wild meat. Here I can't get any."

On a later visit, I was remonstrating with my friend: "Russ you can walk the halls and I'd go on outside with you where you used to go out under the fruit trees. I remember Cullen was sitting up in one, watching you."

"Can't get on my feet without an Aide and then I have to be in one of those damn belts."

"I know, so they can hold on to you, so you won't fall."

"I'd get right back up." Russ boomed. "I'd get right back up!"

"And not stop thinking." I said to myself.

On another visit, I stood at the door of his new room. Another change due to a fight with a roommate. Russ was sleeping; I hated to disturb him but I had a rare Louis L'Amour book. He devoured all of them. Russ sat up, excited about the book and the Event of the day. He'd been with the friend who was taking care of Russ's beloved dog. They both were searching for the animal since it ran away.

"I took his favorite ball and I went two miles. Oh, have you seen my motorized chair, a real go-cart. Well, we called and called. Thought I heard my dog so I threw the ball out. You should see how your idea for my bad hand worked. Well, he must have smelled it and came racing to me, mouth full of ball!"

I gave Russ some Geology papers. "You look them over; I can't figure them out, but they're of places you told me about."

"That's the place named for William Clark's sweetheart. I'll make it there again – can't give up or you're whipped. Oh, a bunch of us went to a fancy restaurant, everything, even shrimp cocktail."

"Ah, did the mountain man go Citicorp?" I teased.

When I started to leave, I looked back to wave; our cowboy was lying on his bed engrossed in geology maps. As our ten-year friendship drew to a close, we visited him at a private home in the country. His eyes gleamed Labrodorite again at the Humming birds in the lush back yard. He told us about going fishing and then, in the autumn hunting with the husband of the Aide who left the Nursing Home to take Russ into their home, giving him the same skilled care. What a miracle! We continued to hear his wild stories and sad ones; the wife who had left him taking their boy with her and both were killed in a car crash.

"No, no chewing gum. I have only one tooth left," he said from his motorized chair sporting a fiendish grin.

He went out on the lawn with that special cowboy set to the shoulders, the good arm bent at the elbow, in a "here-I-am-still-in-the-saddle" statement!

However, our friend could not "get back up" from a cancer that was too determined and won. 1920 to 2008, our special Cowboy!

Harold and Ellie

The mustard-colored hat! I wheeled closer to the wearer and shook hands. He said, "My name's Harold. Glad to meet ya, you betcha."

"I could not take my eyes off your hat and the feathers."

"It's a real Stetson. You betcha! It's old now."

Harold took off his prize hat, showed me the sweat stains. "I was with my daughter's boyfriend in L.A. He'd been in some movies. He took me to the best store and I tried on this hat. Oh, I really wanted it. You betcha I did. Cost too much. Two, three days later, the young fella brought me the hat. Now that was a great son-in-law!"

I agreed. I almost said, "You betcha."

"He's head of the State Police over in Nevada. They're divorced now, but he's a great fella, you betcha."

Harold was from Idaho where his great-uncle was first homesteader in Nemhi County. "There's a creek named after him. I learned horses over there near Salmon, great quarter horses raised up in the hills. My granddad from England knew horses but not like those. Did you ever read about Umatilla? Indian name."

"Yes: he's in the Quarter-horse legend book."

"Daughter is Temple Standard like him, but even faster. I rode her in county fairs everywhere and then at the big tracks in Salt Lake City. You betcha that was the famous Quarter-horse racing of the whole country. Temple Standard was so proud. Big white blaze face, she'd come out of her train car, down the ramp and look around to be sure hundreds of people there to see her. Yep, just to see her! She'd hold her head up high, her ears up. The peg-leg man who owned her, he was a millionaire, he'd let folks know what siding his private horse car would be on. Great horse: I could ride her in two, even three races in one day. She'd breathe hard, you betcha. Her nostrils would be red but hardly bulging. Just loved to run. Loved to see those crowds! Oh you hafta meet my wife. You betcha, meet my wife."

He brought her to the table. Her enigmatic expression said she was glad Harold was explaining things he loved. Ellie smiled; the wide, square nose widened and her eyes crinkled. Ellie – always bent over in her wheel chair, sometimes with the oxygen tubes in her nose form the portable tank attached. She had a wise little look; life was wry and you took whatever was there, it said. She grew up "smack in the dead center of Kansas." Her first husband was a ranch cook so they kept moving further and further west. One day when I talked with her, Ellie was beaming: her granddaughter had visited after she won the Barrel-racing trophy in the Finals of the National Rodeo! The young girl had come from somewhere far away, "so good to see her." Generally, Ellie did not say much about herself. Just how you had to be a worker like her grandmother who "kept house in a homestead soddie."

Harold and Ellie met and married in the Home. As with other couples there, if Ellie was taken to the hospital, Harold would be taken by the facility's van for visits. Sentiment and sense. Then the spouse at the Home was less anxious. Having to go to the hospital hinted at terminal illness. Harold was solicitous about Ellie; he'd gently push her chair indoors and out. No, they didn't share a room. "Ellie has to have oxygen all night," he told me. However, he didn't protest when Ellie wanted to be wheeled to the room for smokers.

From M.T.'s father I learned Harold was well known, not just as a horseman but also as a violinist. He was a steady at the National Landmark Hotel. Tall Harold also had been a brawler, any word about his music or racing that was taken wrong led to a fight. I asked Harold about the music and he bragged about his "fiddle." "Not a Stradivarius but something like it. I've been offered $4,000.00 and more for it. However, I won't sell it; I keep it safe at my daughter's. She's in the hospital business, knows all about finances. My other daughter remarried – into the family that raised elk over in Idaho. You know the big ranch?"

Harold was telling about a son. Proudly, he went on, "Went to funeral director school and has two big places now. Makes a lot of money, my son. He's somewhere in California."

Harold's bony arm gestured, generally west, and his other hand was bandaged. He made no mention of it but Ellie said he had a fight with his roommate. To my amazement, I learned that Ellie fought too. She pulled monitors out, battled the Aides as they tried to put the oxygen tube in her nose and despite many breathing emergencies, Ellie still insisted Harold wheel her into the smoker's room.

Recently I had a dream, one of those vivid videos in the head: A hooded person was racing in a wheelchair down the halls of our Nursing Home. Head and shoulders were bent like a jockey. The chair was going to hit the Day Room furniture and the glass cases with the birds. I braced myself for the crash and for the shrieking of the Finches! But no. The mad racer stopped. The gray hood came down, the head bent over the knees.

Was I thinking of Ellie or Harold, their pent-up desire – Harold on Temple Standard, Ellie proud of her work, Edith leading the sheep or in her room at home, gazing at the Shining Mountains? Or was the mad racer the Cowboy, acting on his desire to get out across to Oregon again. Perhaps M.T. free of crutches, braces and blessed Edwina free – no more slings nor canes – free to stride with her daughter. And M.T. to catch sand dollars. Strange things, dreams of other people's dreams!

Rose

  The next person I came to know was already familiar to me before we met, proving the power of imagination. One October night I heard an emergency announcement on a police scanner. I wrote a poem as I visualized the missing person, nameless, simply an item on a police scanner and the circumstances.

The scanner crackled
As we came in
"Elderly lady wandering"
A naughty sin!   Wandering

I wonder as I wander
Out under the sky
How my man, my true love,
Had come for to die?

She lived alone since –
How long had he been dead?
Her legs were iron, to dare was to walk
A gang plank suspended in air.

They said,
"She didn't even try.
Didn't even turn the key in the truck.
He left her a perfectly good truck!"

Perhaps no small hand in hers,
"Oh, Ma, look!"
Dark eyes intense and bright
Rage of her rage, light of her light.

Only the familiars safe instead,
The myriad worlds within her head.
Until that night she burst
Out of the ranch house door.

Arms wide to the wind
Dark sky,
And walked!
To the ends of the earth!

Not a bad place to walk to or,
As they said and *they* are astute,
Wandered to him,
Buried and mute.

They found her
Chilled, not dead,
And tucked her snug
In a Nursing Home bed.

I passed my poem around and the nurses sent me to a special wing of the Home following my hunch. Her voice was deep and brusque and her head low over the schoolroom type chair with a tray across the front, useful for restraining a patient. I was told Rose was sometimes violent. The dark hair and eyes were just as I pictured.

I quietly said, "My name's June."

Her electric energy flowed with warmth as she said, "That was my mother's name."

Her large rancher's hands had been clenched together on the tray but in that first encounter and all others, Rose eased them apart so I could hold one hand. Her strong grip strengthened me. The last time I sat beside her, a loud speaker buzzed above us. I was so startled, I sputtered a few tears and Rose rebuked me. I needed that. Later I added to the poem:

Nurses say they choose when to die,
But we protest out of guilt,
What will be said of us?
We can depend on their strong knowing.

She could not have bossed the ranch
Without a strong knowing!
If we let the strong ones
Say what tugs at their hearts,

Flex old legs and walk to the end of the earth,
Moving on is a bright awareness
To breathe the great night wind!
Savoring instead of sipping, as free as she went

To her man's wide arms
And held muscle to muscle against his center.
She knew – that autumn night
She strode to the ends of the earth!

Later I searched for Rose's new room. She was comatose. Above her head were precise instructions "Turn every two hours." I moved quietly as if still approaching the Rose of the pent-up energy. I had brought the two parts of the poem, and relatives put it next to Rose's wedding picture in which even "her man" looked as I'd imagined him. There was a big family photo, too; rows of dark-haired folk with square jaws, serious dark eyes, Rose's eyes. All could have been stamped out from the same genetic machine. I was told they were Rose's brothers and sisters.

"And here's a very old picture when the parents first came from Austria," one of the visitors said. "They homesteaded over on the bench."

"Kids bought more land?"

"Yes they did. Then uncles settled over huge areas. You see the family name everywhere. You hear it said two ways. We joke. The ones who raise cows say the hard 'c' at the end, and the ones with sheep say it like 'sh.'"

Rose never saw what I wrote and I'll never know if her family kept the poem.

Edwina

Ten years propped in bed, the last year moved only by means of a Hoyer lift. (I remembered it from the last months of my mother's life after 13 years at our house.) The lift was a crane that moved a sling under the patient's body, which then could be swung sideways from the bed into a wheelchair. Edwina's vehicle was exceptionally large with a high extension up the back to support her head. Like Christopher Reeves, she was pushed about and was fed in this chair, her eyes big and searching about, always luminous. When I first saw Edwina, we talked about her ceiling full of kitten pictures.

I marveled at her glowing skin. I inwardly praised the staff for giving her great care – always clean, fresh hospital gown and bedding. I could only ponder about the work needed for her hygiene, the medical expertise to counter the swelling of her feet and legs, a dangerous complication, plus strokes that further wrecked Edwina, a victim of extreme multiple sclerosis. I learned about compassion as I was near Edwina. Toward the end, nurses told me they almost lost her again. She wanted a drink of water. I saw none on her bedside table.

"No," the Aide warned me, "she might aspirate with water."

"But she wants it so much," said I, the amateur.

"Here, she loves thickened coke."

Caution even after years in a downward spiral. Then I saw a tiny newspaper obituary. Edwina had died. Yes, her daughter was there and a baby granddaughter. There were parents far away in San Diego. But a life of her own? A stroke at age 43 after years of a chronic disease that crept up on her, a lifetime of trouble.

Edwina said she was puzzled why she couldn't move. "Some days worse." She used her hands and her fine mind worked, especially through those great and marvelous eyes. She forced her distorted mouth to form words, and the more I was with her the more natural her speaking seemed to me because we had made a link. We had agreed the physical world was sometimes "a bummer."

"Excuse my slow-ness. The Speech Therapist said I would tire people waiting. On the phone to my mother I thought I sounded weird, my garbled 'He-l-lo'."

"I'm not tiring. I hear your words clearly and I like to talk with you. If you tire, I'll go, Edwina."

"No, Stay! I am not tir-er-ed. Stay and talk."

"Or when you want, I'll watch your TV with you."

Edwina told me when we first met that she watched certain soap-operas. "Just habit."

We talked and talked. I asked about the two photos on the wall: a beautiful baby, sitting up in bed with her arms extended toward a dark-haired woman at the edge of the picture. Her face was fixed on the child as if she couldn't get her fill.

"My baby, Monica, at six months. She's going to be a senior in High School now, over six feet tall. Wants to be a model." Edwina worried about her daughter's plans to go to New York City for the summer. The Nursing staff allowed Edwina to use the office phone so she had frequent calls from her mother, the grandmother, who had taken Monica to a California boarding school. Soon after I met Edwina, Monica returned to the hometown to start her last high school year and even confided in Edwina; "Yes, there was a boyfriend she had been living with but that was over."

Edwina's eyes glowed, "Monica really wanted to talk. And she really liked my slogan for us: It's rough; hang tough."

"That's what mothers are for."

Even at a distance, Edwina's big and I considered beautiful face had a sideways smile, sidelong from irony, not just the stroke. Lying in bed so much or slumped in her special chair, Edwina's body had become slack; she had a large, brave ampleness, not old when one looked at the wise, full face and the eyes. She knew I knew truths we could not verbalize.

Several people in the Nursing Home told me that when Monica 'blew into' the town, still a teenager, she had grown up too fast; her heavy make-up, the tall model look and that she ran with a fast crowd. Edwina spoke of Monica's father and how they lived in his mountain cabin when they were still a family. Some said he took Monica back up there. Then the change back to the boarding school, and it was the father who arranged for Monica to spend Christmas back in the town where the Nursing Home was. Edwina was joyous afterward. Mother and daughter had long, warm talks. Again, Edwina felt like a needed person!

"And yes, I'm missing her, but I know how my parents must have felt when I went back to boarding school after holidays at home. I lived near Balboa Park there in San Diego. Great gardens there. I'd walk and walk..."

Edwina's life had been a series of Quaker boarding schools in Canada and Oregon and then college on the West Coast. "...the rush, the buildings; I decided there must be a better life somewhere besides L.A."

"Then you came here to the mountains?"

"That won't take long to tell." Her speech slowed, "Tha—t won't be- com-pli-ca-ted."

"We'll leave it to next time? Yes? Edwina?"

"Y-e-s."

However, Edwina only answered with the smile when I came to her bedside the next day. "How did I come to be here?" A long pause and then she laughed. "You can – see I still here."

We talked of many things, my worry-topic, a little grandson who was a special needs child. Edwina's wisdom shone through those brown eyes: "He's taking it slowly. It is a scary world out there."

I met Edwina's adoptive parents when they traveled from San Diego to see her. The mother had been an English war bride. "Oh, we two met on a train, mind you. He was such a bonny soldier!"

The father was serious, told me he was an engineer in West Coast research. I knew I could not inquire, as I often wanted to when visiting Edwina: Why wasn't she in a California nursing complex? My contact with her parents was cut short; they were called back. Their adopted son (Edwina spoke of him as being unstable) had an accident, had a nervous breakdown and was being brought to their house.

Not to be crass, but I was reminded of an old Yiddish saying about "tsouris." Test a group of people; have each one put his/her problems into a separate basket and then give each a choice of which troubles basket to exchange for one's own. Each person would take back his/her own basket of "tsouris."

So for my observations of Edwina, I do not use her real name; her husband's family might resent my revelations. Perhaps they should know her life history. Perhaps they never knew the extensive medical catastrophes she had. I visited with Edwina for nine years after we were together in the Home. There was a haunting peacefulness in her private room where nurses came in to move Edwina in her bed or into her huge special wheelchair to take her to the dining room for the most disabled clients. There an Aide, often the most skilled ex-Army medic, fed her. Thomas was so respectful of Edwina. She would grin as she candidly declared Thomas more handsome than the 'lover-boy' in one of the 'TV Soaps.' Edwina, a young soul crying out of those wise, huge eyes and caught in an immobile body slowly, slowly dying.

Perhaps her husband's family *did* know, were secretly helping to cover for his absence. Or was it all more com-pli-ca-ted, than anyone, especially Edwina, could say? I respect the discretion of the Nursing Home staff. They knew my closeness to her. Over the years of visits, I never probed and no one revealed how she came to be in our area. Edwina talked with her head propped but her body slumped and I longed to lean over the bedrail and shift her, but her neck and shoulder muscles were weakening.

"It all began when I was 22, just coming into bloom," Edwina was telling me.

"There was a tingling in my arms, then suddenly one leg would not support me, I was hurrying to get dressed for to work. 'What's going on,' I asked the Doctor. He took tests, asked me a hundred questions and the next week he said, 'I'm sorry to have to tell you but you have Multiple Sclerosis, M.S.' 'What's that'?"

Edwina continued, "He said it did not mean the end of the world, just you'll have to do things differently – no more dance classes, get help some times. HA! I told him that it wouldn't be...," she choked.

I said, "Wouldn't be the end of *his* world!"

She gave me one of her deep, shattering glances agreeing.

I looked over the photos of Edwina and the baby. "They're like action pictures: you smiling, the next one you're open-mouthed and the baby's almost bouncing from the bed. The little turned up nose. She's a delightful little elf!"

Edwina brought us back to the present, to Monica's being at a new boarding school.

"She must be all right. If she was miserable, she'd call her grandparents to take her home."

"Will she come here again for Christmas and good talks again?"

"She's a good kid, yes."

Edwina told me she'd been "Trundled to the Doctor, fluid building up so I'm to have that – you know, *that* – everyday."

"The whirlpool?"

"That's it! It is wonderful. I love it."

Monica had written a poem or copied it from some book at school. "She's not the poetic type, but this has many outdoor descriptions. Maybe she thinks Nature is kind."

I could feel the need for release, need of a storm as Edwina blurted out, "Nature is NOT kind!" She struggled but untangled her arm from the pillows and lifted it to say, "I'm shaking it at God!"

"There's a play on Broadway now: *My Arms Aren't Long Enough To Box With God*," I told her.

"Are we called patients here because we are patient? I've been patient long enough!"

I found myself shaking my arm, too and then slipped into the habit of preachyness words I often use for my storms. I told Edwina, "God's clearer to us when we get mad and argue with Him."

"Yes, that – is – true." Edwina was tiring. Her words were stretching out.

One afternoon as we talked, we heard music. Edwina was excited. "Someone is celebrating, maybe a birthday!" she blurted out loudly. "I feel like going there. Let's party!"

I found the call bell. The wire had fallen down the side of her guardrail. We could hear it buzzing at the nurse's station down the hall. How often I felt for the nurses when the buzzing and the lights above patients' doors interfered with their constant paperwork. But an RN came in cheerfully, everyone was fond of and reacted to Edwina's graciousness, and the process was set in motion. Two Aides, the sling, the huge wheelchair and down to the festival we went.

"My birthday was just eight days ago," Edwina told me as she pulled a card out of her pocket. A loving message '...from Mom and Dad.' Was it the only card? I didn't ask, only wished I'd known.

I thought of my lone Christmas card on Altha Mae's bulletin board. But we rolled on faster – "I see a really big cake! We'll live it up!"

Later, in her room again, Edwina and I looked at the silent snow beginning to fall, I thought of my long drive back to my home.

Her eyes and mine locked. "It's a scary world out there," Edwina said slowly.

Oh, I so hoped she did not think I regretted being there. How could I tell her I longed for a miracle, for her to rise up, able to pick up her pallet and walk away from the years of misery? She knew. Then we both were drawn to the winter gray. The silence. The haunting desire to draw the walls in around us and retreat form the scary world forever. The snowflakes veiled the coming darkness.

On a later visit, a momentary chill came between us. I was in the assisted-feeding area. I remembered the times I'd wheel in beside her when she was being fed by the favorite Aide she'd flirtatiously declared more handsome than a movie actor. Now I was looking in from the outside, even driving about, a visitor. I didn't want to stare at the dish of sauce being spooned to her, so I stepped apart from Edwina to bend over Rose, the ranch lady of my poem. Her head was bent over the food tray. I spoke my name, reminding Rose how it was the same as her mother's, so she would not resist looking up but perhaps warm to familiar words. Quickly I looked across at Edwina. Did I imagine a strange expression or was I foolishly thinking I looked like "Lady Bountiful," the stereotype of the volunteer visitor bestowing momentary babble right and left? Did she think I was not truly her friend? That very day I'd been the busy body when mail from a Quaker foundation had arrived for Edwina. The delivery Volunteer had questioned it; I explained firmly that Edwina had attended Quaker schools and she must still have contacts. But that moment and her expression in the dining room. Was our bond fragile? Especially now that I was an outsider?

One has to rest in the truth. And we learn from wise ones, like Altha Mae. I remember her words: "Inner minds understand each other." Altha told me once, "Sometimes we worry that we did or said something a friend has misapplied. How we worry. We think about our ways a day or two. Then time clears it all. True friends know what transpired was all right."

So another patient I had come to love became, through her comforting wisdom, part of the inter-connectedness. Is it because we met inside? A place where we were not a-flutter in busy-ness that we were able to bond, talk and were free of responsibilities? Perhaps we were like Plato's philosophers with only thinking as their daily task. I hate to conclude the only way inner minds connected, but let us list this opportunity as one more aspect, and a most favorable one, of life *FROM THE INSIDE.*

Sand Dollars – M. T.

She asked me to write about a happier time; there were not many – oh, some while teaching on the Reservation, but the day of the sand dollars was unique and symbolic. More than that, it involved M.T.'s brother, Bud.

"We were at Coos Bay with our folks and we found a small, special beach. I don't know if it had a name but we had it all to ourselves, Bud and me. The Oregon surf was really up and we were excited to see the spray tossing up sand dollars! If you didn't catch them, they'd fall and be pulled out to sea."

M.T. continued, "I had my camera. I was using crutches then and I moved out into the wet sand as Jim leaped up. I snapped a picture of him, feet off the ground. It was wonderful: against the sky, the water iridescent. The perfect moment! Suddenly I realized my crutches were being sucked down into the wet sand."

"Save the camera, don't worry about me! Just save the camera! And he did. You have to catch moments, any bits of treasure tossed up before the surf can pull them back and the magic is gone."

Even when the wet sand threatens to suck your crutches down into the surf...M.T. lives on, alone now and, miracle of miracles, taking care of herself. Five years ago, she painted the picture of the sand dollars from the magic photograph.

M.T. seemed young when I first met her at what her father called "the Rest Home." She walked carefully, leaning on a high walker, forearms resting on the tray on top. Meds and sketchpad were in a basket clipped to the legs of the walker. Maybe she seemed younger because of her quaint, long dresses worn to cover leg braces and the awkward, heavy shoes. Since M.T. is an artist, the dresses were lovely, Empire waist, stylish prints and wonderful colors. Yes, she was like a child as she spread peanut butter and jelly on her bread.

"Most foods disagree with me," she explained. "Due to the many stomach surgeries."

I always remember how she'd lick the remaining jelly from the corners of the small containers. All of us at the *Board of Directors* table would slide our restaurant-type jelly pats to M.T. Her golden-brown eyes sparkled. Yes, golden-brown, sometimes sloe-eyed as she'd lean forward over the high walker, fingering the one long plait of her wavy hair that hung over one shoulder. We always exchanged eye glances during meals and as she rose to return to her room. She needed her lung-cleaning nebulizer.

I would knock and then wheel in, squeezing my wheelchair in between boxes, high trays piled with art supplies, magazines, and rubber-banded bundles of medical bills.

"I've sold two more paintings! That will help pay some of the bills!" M.T. announced. She was an award-winning painter.

As spring and summer came, M.T. would line up photographs of the previous year's plantings; they looked like calendar pictures of English gardens. Her father, age 83, was in charge of the town's landscaping – a vigorous, handsome man, eager to tell anyone who'd stop about his World War II exploits. M.T.'s seemingly sane mother would take her to their house some afternoons so she could plant blooms in their garden, M.T. using a long handled hoe as she leaned on her high walker. Soon her room was overwhelmed with cut flowers and I longed to ask for some as she and I labored twice a day in P.T., but I didn't want to interrupt her; she was diligent, braces and all.

For a while, M.T. had lived her dream: to teach Indian children after she graduated college with honors in two majors. She took a job as Art/English teacher and Librarian at a Reservation in the bleak part of her state. It was windswept land and cold. M.T. lived in a trailer.

"I closed off two rooms. They'd freeze. I hardly needed a fridge. But I was late for classes only once!"

"How did you make it out?" they'd ask.

"I shoveled, dug my car out. Didn't have crutches then."

All day she taught both subjects and then her time after school was spent ordering or cataloging the library books and repairing the many old ones. And always the children! How to get them to read and get the right books for them. M.T.'s fragile health broke. Back home, in and out of hospitals, she painted the faces of "her" Indian children, especially a 4th grade boy she worried about.

He was so bright, a mind as fleeting as the sand dollars, capturing learning but the magic would recede as he was pushed off to one relative or another. His common-law parents did not qualify[15] for a house on the Reservation and they often were not even in their heatless wreck of a trailer nearby.

But M.T. struggled in her own way, keeping the child in her drawings, haunting and in her heart. She longed to bring him home but she had no place of her own and her mother seemed to want to be closer; took art classes with M.T., 'into flowers' as the townspeople put it. M.T. herself was accepted as a special student of a nationally known artist, and was named *Artist of the Year*. Her work was exhibited at galleries and at her college. She was commissioned to illustrate novels about the history of her area and her own nature subjects, leaves of dramatic Canadian Maple trees and of curled Sycamore were symbols of stirring emotions with the shapes, the full patterns and shadows. Her controlled watercolors impressed buyers.

But she had more surgeries, more travel to specialists and to larger hospitals out-of-state. M.T. had been sickly as a child, missing months of school so friendships were few and tenuous. Oh, family friends, her roots went far back in the town, made murmurs of praise about M.T. "bravely pushing that high walker down the aisle at church" and her art work but she

---

[15] Tribal authenticity.

said, "I call my friends; so many went off to jobs but some have come back."

"And they...?" I had not seen many visitors.

"They come over, some of them."

M.T. spoke of going out to dinner; I hoped with old school friends, but later it slipped out that she had gone with her parents.

"Friends say they'd like to take me places but then they back out. 'Don't know how you'd get in the car.' OH, I was so excited when two of them said maybe I could come along to Celebration Days at the ghost town. I love that place and one of the two has permission to stay overnight at the old hotel."

I held my breath. Something told me M.T. did not go.

"They called back and said maybe I'd fall on the old broken sidewalks. They went on over."

Worse was the refusal of Jim's, "...my closest friend, way back even in grade school. Oh, not a boyfriend. I wish I had one," as tears came to M.T.'s eyes. I had never seen her cry about anything. "Jim's doing well in his business and said he'd help me with anything – legal things."

"Could your dad – or your mother help?"

"Dad's getting old. He tried. And mother..."

The trouble was brewing between them and her mother couldn't keep her own affairs or bills in order. M.T. explained this to Jim. "Is she seeing a doctor?" Jim was wriggling out of his offer. "What does your brother say?"

"Oh, Jim, he's only seen her once; the last time he was here for only one week. He thinks we're overreacting. Besides tranquilizers and anti-depressants are supposed to work."

Jim felt the warning signs, heard the rumors. "You know, I just can't get involved. Look, our mothers go 'way back.' It would just make more trouble."

Other friends, lawyers went back, so M.T. pushed her grief inside but when she was discharged from the nursing home, the van left her at the house one afternoon her father was away. He volunteered at the History Museum. Her mother greeted her strangely and then stood over her, closer and closer. M.T. moved her walker and pulled herself toward the portable phone but her mother, now glaring, pushed her against the wall. M.T. had just managed to grab the phone and as she fell, she curled her fingers around it as her mother's hands pressed against her neck, pressing hard at her throat. Quickly M.T. inched her body away, farther and farther as her mother released the hold and rushed to her bedroom. There were sounds of things being thrown. Later they saw that all the clothes had been pulled off hangers, all dresser items smashed. M.T. finally heard the door slam and her mother's car roar away.

Counselors were appointed but the mother appeared at only one session. She stood at the office doorway and then dashed away after telling M.T. she despised her. Sunk in the chair across form the psychologist who in many meetings had been so kind to her, M.T. said, "What can I do? We loved each other so much."

"You've tried. We all have. That's all we can do."

"What can I pay you with?" M.T. asked at their last session.

"A painting." The Counselor replied. "Yes, one of your watercolors would be my best reward."

"I'll do a new one. What do you like? A Place? A still life of…?"

"The sea. I grew up on the Oregon coast. I miss the colors of the ocean."

M.T. was excited, " Oregon! Coos Bay! My family and I were there once and there were sand dollars…"

As M.T. told me about their choice for the painting and the coincidence, she glowed young again, shoulder pulled up like a biker setting off. Off on a road trip she could never venture on except through her painting of the sand dollars caught in the surf.

June A. W. Severance

My Last Roommate

One afternoon I was approached about changing rooms just as I was wheeling rapidly to attend Mass. The Priest came only infrequently. I liked the cozy room I'd been in for less than a week after I'd been returned from the intensive care at the hospital. The Social Services people persisted; I persisted, Mass was starting.

"I feel like I'm in a Motel," I burbled.

"We just wanted to give you a choice. A person is coming to the other bed – a very interesting person, been all over the world, loves books. You could stay in your present room with this roommate."

This sounded like the sales pitch when admitting my father long ago. I just rattled, "Fine. Fine."

Actually, I had seen this person the evening before. Fred B. had a visitor and he did introduce me in his courtly way, saying they'd been talking about Holland.

I joined in about how I'd like the Netherlands from the first views from the train. "Felt I'd been there before, the scenes were living pictures by artists I liked."

The stranger agreed in a Dutch accent and a pleasant smile. I was pleased Fred had a guest, perhaps Fred knew from his travels, maybe took photos in Holland. I did notice the visitor's long dress, but what about the deep voice, the face that needed a shave?

Returning to "my" room; after Mass, I saw an array of satin slips and bras, a housecoat with ruffles. The theatrical curtains were abruptly closed to surround the bed across the room, as the facility's rules were clear: "It is important to respect the space of one's bed area and that of the occupant of the other bed and bed stand." The nurse, one of two on each wing on day shift, one at night, arrived and conversed behind the cyclorama, the drapes around the other bed. The deep voice answering the nurse's questions was the same, the same Dutch accent as Fred's guest. But the Individual was becoming angry.

"I WANT to see my doctor. NOW!"

"Only when he makes rounds once a week or so. This is not your hospital surgical floor," the nurse reasoned with the patient.

The Individual brought up more problems, like demanding trays for breakfast and lunch. This was against rules and against the best re-habilitation procedures; post-surgical patients need to move about. The next day an Aide, my delightful buddy, Faye, gently announced to the curtained-off-bed that patients were to be in the dining room in 5 or 10 minutes. "Would you like me to bring in a wheelchair and help you?"

A deep roar thundered! I was sitting on the side of my bed as vitals were being taken and the electronic thermometer popped out of my mouth. I think the vibrations were about to send me bouncing off the bed as the deep voice yelled.

"Sorry I asked!" The usually calm and loving Faye flounced out. So touching, she returned later to apologize to the Individual, my term for the him that became a her.

We talked that night from bed to bed about books, about his/her teaching college chemistry in Europe.

I asked, "How did you come to live in America?"

"Our minister preached in USA and he recruited us to return with him."

"And how did you come here?"

"Just us, traveled all over America. An opening just for a while came up and we stayed."

I did not want to pry just whom the "we" meant. A wife? Or a travel companion? I was not in the room much, avoided it during the day with two times in P.T. again. I couldn't believe how muscles became limp in the forced lack of movement at the hospital where I had to "fake" out the blood clots. I liked visiting all the friends and I admit I felt a weird tingling whenever I was dressing or just being in the room with the Individual. Now I did not dislike the person, just that I retreated to the bathroom, which, as the male Aides always said, "Gives you some privacy."

One night a Registered Nurse and I were together for a procedure and the male Aide who'd helped me out of bed began talking with us. We three were being inconsiderate but we were just used to chatting.

From the curtained bed came the LOUD DUTCH roars. "Give me a different room. Now! Medjelty. I go! I go this moment!"

The nurse and Aide slunk away. I pulled the blankets over my ears as even the window curtains quivered.

The Individual's charm beamed at everyone at evening meals and at music programs. Truly, my roommate dressed splendidly, strode along with flowing long skirts. One time I attempted to wheel along but suddenly thunder and lightning clattered past me in fashionable high heels but bare, very male ankles. The strong, boney face was distraught. Had I committed some offense?

The staff had known the Individual from previous stays at the Nursing Home but they discreetly told nothing of the circumstances. A fellow resident revealed simply that a professor was known to have gone to have a sex change. The man had been labeled a Transvestite upon first coming to the area. No leer. No editorializing.

Then on my last evening, our talk became personal about the future. "I have no one. Back where I live, I must go to taking care of myself all alone. Sometimes I am very sick," the Individual's voice was mournful.

I said words of sympathy, but they seemed clichés. I knew so little of the person's true being. I was feeling naïve like a pampered child because I had a loved one, a happy home, grandchildren, friends —

including all those at the Home I'd come to love. My roommate said there was no one to talk to. The deep voice spoke again.

"I hope you achieve what you wish."

There was a very knowing edge to that statement, as we each understood there were secrets we knew and chose not to verbalize as we said goodbye.

June A. W. Severance

Departures and Goodbyes

Farewells came soon, too soon while I was at the Home.

Each morning I'd call out to Elsie when her wheelchair approached and I would see her sweet face. Not a false, saccharine sweetness, just a light in her pale face with its halo of white hair. Elsie warmed to everyone, wheeling up with a word about each person's feelings, sad or happy. Moving took effort, her one good arm worked one wheel of her chair and her feet paddled on the floor to keep it going.

However, I knew, even before the Social Director came over to tell me that Elsie had passed away. No more, "How are you, Elsie?"

"I'm fine, I'm fine. And you?"

"We'll all miss that...her smile."

But no chance to say, "Goodbye! Farewell!"

Saying Goodbyes takes me back to Norma, my sophisticated California friend. When I visited her for years after I was discharged, she would grin and pop off some risqué joke like a skilled, stand-up comedian. Those obsidian eyes always glinting. She no longer kept up the illusion of eventually living permanently in her son's house. I had been so know-it-all, thinking it cruel that Norma was being fooled – as if she could ever be strung along. Instead, she enjoyed some weekends there, most holidays, and she triumphed over winning at dominoes with her youngest great-grandchild.

Norma still loved smart clothes and spoke like my family of years past when she commented favorably if I was wearing something smart, a true Chicago term to me. I praised her well-matched outfits. I teased Norma about her dozens of shoes bulging from the shoe-bag hung outside her closet. "Just call me Mrs. Marcos!"

Norma was excited over the latest publicity photo-shot of her grandson on location in Mexico. "To think my baby grand-boy has been in films for twenty-five years!"

We agreed about good genes as we hugged goodbye. "Love you!" she always called out.

I ran into Norma in a Radiation facility waiting room. Her hair was disheveled. Usually Norma had a weekly appointment with the excellent Beautician at the Nursing Home. It was strange, too, to see her in a colorless hospital robe; there was always a glow from her bright blouses. Norma's face was pale and very gaunt.

"I've just been to my son's. Oh! It's lovely there in my suite with my hot tub. I could loll there forever. In the suite, not the tub. It makes me a lobster."

The Texas twang, still some of the wit but the California style was just a whisper.

"But then I might not. There's something wrong with my insides – ugly words and nasty place to take treatments. You know, I'll wreck the camera."

I almost topped her words with some crack about "You always wanted to be in pictures."

Could she still take our jokes? This gal from a hard-scrabble farm, the single mom who marched up to the bank every payday, depositing enough for a "real west coast house for my kids!" A nurse came for her so Norma and I hugged gently. She seemed to evaporate right in front of me. I knew it was a last goodbye. "Love ya" and Norma tipped her head and waved. "Let the cameras roll!"

June A. W. Severance

The End

Biography
June A. W. Severance

Child stage performer, Chicago, including World's Fair – 1933

MA from Syracuse University, New York. Taught in English Department.

Worked as Women's News Editor broadcasting Daily Radio Programs WKZO (CBS affiliate) Michigan.

Edited Newspaper: American Association of University Women, St. Louis, Missouri.

Fifty years as lecturer/One Woman shows: books, authors: lives, reviews of Broadway plays and interviews with cast members.

Wrote/produced shows for Fisher Price Co. East Aurora, New York. Directed plays for professional and community theaters in Midwest and New York State.

Preformed her own prose and poetry at Arts Humanities Center, Virginia City, Montana

She met her beloved husband in 1946. They have 2 sons and 5 grand-children.

June A. W. Severance

APPENDIX

State Regulations Pertaining to Resident Rights[16]

Federal Regulations

Resident rights.

The resident has a right to a dignified existence, self-determination, and communication with and access to persons and services inside and outside the facility. A facility must protect and promote the rights of each resident, including each of the following rights:

(a) Exercise of rights.

(1) The resident has the right to exercise his or her rights as a resident of the facility and as a citizen or resident of the United States.

(2) The resident has the right to be free of interference, coercion, discrimination, and reprisal from the facility in exercising his or her rights.

(3) In the case of a resident adjudged incompetent under the laws of a State by a court of competent jurisdiction, the rights of the resident are exercised by the person appointed under State law to act on the resident's behalf.

(4) In the case of a resident who has not been adjudged incompetent by the State court, any

---

[16] **Resident Rights State and Federal Regulations**
http://www.hpm.umn.edu/nhregsplus/NH%20Regs%20by%20Topic/NH%20Regs%20Topic%20Pdfs/Resident%20Rights/category_resident_rights_FINAL.pdf

legal-surrogate designated in accordance with State law may exercise the resident's rights to the extent provided by State law.

(b) Notice of rights and services. 300 of 306 09/11/07

State Regulations pertaining to category_resident_rights

Federal Regulations

(1) The facility must inform the resident both orally and in writing in a language that the resident understands of his or her rights and all rules and regulations governing resident conduct and responsibilities during the stay in the facility. The facility must also provide the resident with the notice (if any) of the State developed under section 1919(e)(6) of the Act. Such notification must be made prior to or upon admission and during the resident's stay. Receipt of such information, and any amendments to it, must be acknowledged in writing;

(2) The resident or his or her legal representative has the right — (i) Upon an oral or written request, to access all records pertaining to himself or herself including current clinical records within 24 hours (excluding weekends and holidays); and (ii) After receipt of his or her records for inspection, to purchase at a cost not to exceed the community standard photocopies of the records or any portions of them upon request and 2 working days advance notice to the facility.

(3) The resident has the right to be fully informed in language that he or she can understand of his or her total health status, including but not limited to, his or her medical condition;

(4) The resident has the right to refuse treatment, to refuse to participate in experimental research, and to formulate an advance directive as specified in paragraph (8) of this section; and

(5) The facility must — (i) Inform each resident who is entitled to Medicaid benefits, in writing, at the time of admission to the nursing facility or, when the resident becomes eligible for Medicaid of —

(A) The items and services that are included in nursing facility services under the State plan and for which the resident may not be charged;

(B) Those other items and services that the facility offers and for which the resident may be charged, and the amount of charges for those services; and (ii) Inform each resident when changes are made to the items and services specified in paragraphs (5)(i) (A) and (B) of this section.

(6) The facility must inform each resident before, or at the time of admission, and periodically during the resident's stay, of services available in the facility and of charges for those services, including any charges for services not covered under Medicare or by the facility's per diem rate.

(7) The facility must furnish a written description of legal rights which includes — (i) A description of the manner of protecting personal funds, under paragraph (c) of this section; (ii) A description of the requirements and procedures for establishing eligibility for Medicaid, including the right to request an assessment under section 1924(c) which determines the extent of a couple's non-exempt resources at the time of institutionalization and attributes to the community spouse an equitable share of resources which cannot be considered available for payment toward the cost of the

institutionalized spouse's medical care in his or her process of spending down to Medicaid eligibility levels; (iii) A posting of names, addresses, and telephone numbers of all pertinent 301 of 306 09/11/07 State Regulations pertaining to category resident rights Federal Regulations State client advocacy groups such as the State survey and certification agency, the State licensure office, the State ombudsman program, the protection and advocacy network, and the Medicaid fraud control unit; and (iv) A statement that the resident may file a complaint with the State survey and certification agency concerning resident abuse, neglect, misappropriation of resident property in the facility, and non-compliance with the advance directives requirements.

(8) The facility must comply with the requirements specified in subpart I of part 489 of this chapter relating to maintaining written policies and procedures regarding advance directives. These requirements include provisions to inform and provide written information to all adult residents concerning the right to accept or refuse medical or surgical treatment and, at the individual's option, formulate an advance directive. This includes a written description of the facility's policies to implement advance directives and applicable State law. Facilities are permitted to contract with other entities to furnish this information but are still legally responsible for ensuring that the requirements of this section are met. If an adult individual is incapacitated at the time of admission and is unable to receive information (due to the incapacitating condition or a mental disorder) or articulate whether or not he or she has executed an advance directive, the facility may give advance

directive information to the individual's family or surrogate in the same manner that it issues other materials about policies and procedures to the family of the incapacitated individual or to a surrogate or other concerned persons in accordance with State law. The facility is not relieved of its obligation to provide this information to the individual once he or she is no longer incapacitated or unable to receive such information. Follow-up procedures must be in place to provide the information to the individual directly at the appropriate time.

(9) The facility must inform each resident of the name, specialty, and way of contacting the physician responsible for his or her care.

(10) The facility must prominently display in the facility written information, and provide to residents and applicants for admission oral and written information about how to apply for and use Medicare and Medicaid benefits, and how to receive refunds for previous payments covered by such benefits.

(11) Notification of changes. (i) A facility must immediately inform the resident; consult with the resident's physician; and if known, notify the resident's legal representative or an interested family member when there is —

(A) An accident involving the resident which results in injury and has the potential for requiring physician intervention;

(B) A significant change in the resident's physical, mental, or psychosocial status (i.e., a deterioration in health, mental, or psychosocial status in either life-threatening conditions or clinical complications);

(C) A need to alter treatment significantly (i.e., a need to discontinue an existing form of treatment due to adverse consequences, or to commence a new form of treatment); or

(D) A decision to transfer or discharge the resident from the facility as specified in § 483.12(a). (ii) The facility must also promptly notify the resident and, if known, the resident's legal representative or interested family member when there is—

(A) A change in room or roommate assignment as specified in § 483.15(e)(2);or

(B) A change in resident rights under Federal or State law or regulations as specified in paragraph (b)(1) of this section. 302 of 306 09/11/07 State Regulations pertaining to category resident rights Federal Regulations (iii) The facility must record and periodically update the address and phone number of the resident's legal representative or interested family member.

(c) **Protection of resident funds.**

(1) The resident has the right to manage his or her financial affairs, and the facility may not require residents to deposit their personal funds with the facility.

(2) Management of personal funds. Upon written authorization of a resident, the facility must hold, safeguard, manage, and account for the personal funds of the resident deposited with the facility, as specified in paragraphs (c)(3)–(8) of this section.

(3) Deposit of funds. (i) Funds in excess of $50. The facility must deposit any residents' personal funds in excess of $50 in an interest bearing account (or accounts) that is separate from any of the facility's operating accounts, and that credits all interest earned

on resident's funds to that account. (In pooled accounts, there must be a separate accounting for each resident's share.) (ii) Funds less than $50. The facility must maintain a resident's personal funds that do not exceed $50 in a noninterest bearing account, interest-bearing account, or petty cash fund.

(4) Accounting and records. The facility must establish and maintain a system that assures a full and complete and separate accounting, according to generally accepted accounting principles, of each resident's personal funds entrusted to the facility on the resident's behalf. (i) The system must preclude any commingling of resident funds with facility funds or with the funds of any person other than another resident. (ii) The individual financial record must be available through quarterly statements and on request to the resident or his or her legal representative.

(5) Notice of certain balances. The facility must notify each resident that receives Medicaid benefits — (i) When the amount in the resident's account reaches $200 less than the SSI resource limit for one person, specified in section 1611(a)(3)(B) of the Act; and (ii) That, if the amount in the account, in addition to the value of the resident's other nonexempt resources, reaches the SSI resource limit for one person, the resident may lose eligibility for Medicaid or SSI.

(6) Conveyance upon death. Upon the death of a resident with a personal fund deposited with the facility, the facility must convey within 30 days the resident's funds, and a final accounting of those funds, to the individual or probate jurisdiction administering the resident's estate.

(7) Assurance of financial security. The facility must purchase a surety bond, or otherwise

provide assurance satisfactory to the Secretary, to assure the security of all personal funds of residents deposited with the facility.

(8) Limitation on charges to personal funds. The facility may not impose a charge against the personal funds of a resident for any item or service for which payment is made under Medicaid or Medicare (except for applicable deductible and coinsurance amounts). The facility may charge the resident for requested services that are more expensive than or in excess of covered services in accordance with § 489.32 of this chapter. (This does not affect the prohibition on facility charges for items and services for which Medicaid has paid. See § 447.15, which limits participation in the Medicaid program to providers who accept, as payment in full, Medicaid payment plus any deductible, coinsurance, or copayment required by the plan to be paid by the individual.) 303 of 306 09/11/07 State Regulations pertaining to category_resident_rights Federal Regulations (i) Services included in Medicare or Medicaid payment. During the course of a covered Medicare or Medicaid stay, facilities may not charge a resident for the following categories of items and services:

(A) Nursing services as required at § 483.30 of this subpart.

(B) Dietary services as required at § 483.35 of this subpart.

(C) An activities program as required at § 483.15(f) of this subpart.

(D) Room/bed maintenance services.

(E) Routine personal hygiene item and services as required to meet the needs of residents, including, but not limited to, hair hygiene supplies, comb, brush, bath soap, disinfecting soaps or specialized cleansing agents when indicated to treat special skin problems or to fight infection, razor, shaving cream, toothbrush, toothpaste, denture adhesive, denture cleaner, dental floss, moisturizing lotion, tissues, cotton balls, cotton swabs, deodorant, incontinence care and supplies, sanitary napkins and related supplies, towels, washcloths, hospital gowns, over the counter drugs, hair and nail hygiene services, bathing, and basic personal laundry.

(F) Medically-related social services as required at § 483.15(g) of this subpart.

(ii) Items and services that may be charged to residents' funds. Listed below are general categories and examples of items and services that the facility may charge to residents' funds if they are requested by a resident, if the facility informs the resident that there will be a charge, and if payment is not made by Medicare or Medicaid:

(A) Telephone.

(B) Television/radio for personal use.

(C) Personal comfort items, including smoking materials, notions and novelties, and confections.

(D) Cosmetic and grooming items and services in excess of those for which payment is made under Medicaid or Medicare.

(E) Personal clothing.

(F) Personal reading matter.

(G) Gifts purchased on behalf of a resident.

(H) Flowers and plants.

(I) Social events and entertainment offered outside the scope of the activities program, provided under § 483.15(f) of this subpart.

(J) Noncovered special care services such as privately hired nurses or Aides.

(K) Private room, except when therapeutically required (for example, isolation for infection control).

(L) Specially prepared or alternative food requested instead of the food generally prepared by the facility, as required by § 483.35 of this subpart.

(iii) Requests for items and services.

(A) The facility must not charge a resident (or his or her representative) for any item or service not requested by the resident.

(B) The facility must not require a resident (or his or her representative) to request any item or service as a condition of admission or continued stay.

(C) The facility must inform the resident (or his or her representative) requesting an item or service for which a charge will be made that there will be a charge for the item or service and what the charge will be.

(d) **Free choice.**

The resident has the right to—304 of 306 09/11/07

State   Regulations   pertaining   to category_resident_rights

Federal Regulations

(1) Choose a personal attending physician;

(2) Be fully informed in advance about care and treatment and of any changes in that care or treatment that may affect the resident's well-being; and

(3) Unless adjudged incompetent or otherwise found to be incapacitated under the laws of the State, participate in planning care and treatment or changes in care and treatment.

(e) **Privacy and confidentiality.**

The resident has the right to personal privacy and confidentiality of his or her personal and clinical records.

(1) Personal privacy includes accommodations, medical treatment, written and telephone communications, personal care, visits, and meetings of family and resident groups, but this does not require the facility to provide a private room for each resident;

(2) Except as provided in paragraph (e)(3) of this section, the resident may approve or refuse the release of personal and clinical records to any individual outside the facility;

(3) The resident's right to refuse release of personal and clinical records does not apply

when — (i) The resident is transferred to another health care institution; or (ii) Record release is required by law.

(f) **Grievances.** A resident has the right to —

(1) Voice grievances without discrimination or reprisal. Such grievances include those with respect to treatment which has been furnished as well as that which has not been furnished; and

(2) Prompt efforts by the facility to resolve grievances the resident may have, including those with respect to the behavior of other residents.

(g) **Examination of survey results.**

A resident has the right to —

(1) Examine the results of the most recent survey of the facility conducted by Federal or State surveyors and any plan of correction in effect with respect to the facility. The facility must make the results available for examination in a place readily accessible to residents, and must post a notice of their availability; and

(2) Receive information from agencies acting as client advocates, and be afforded the
opportunity to contact these agencies.

(h) **Work.**

The resident has the right to—

(1) Refuse to perform services for the facility;

(2) Perform services for the facility, if he or she chooses, when—(i) The facility has documented the need or desire for work in the plan of care; (ii) The plan specifies the nature of the services performed and whether the services are voluntary or paid; (iii) Compensation for paid services is at or above prevailing rates; and (iv) The resident agrees to the work arrangement described in the plan of care.

(i) **Mail.**

The resident has the right to privacy in written communications, including the
right to—

(1) Send and promptly receive mail that is unopened; and

(2) Have access to stationery, postage, and writing implements at the resident's own expense.

(j) **Access and visitation rights.**

305 of 306 09/11/07

State Regulations pertaining to category_resident_rights

Federal Regulations

(1) The resident has the right and the facility must provide immediate access to any resident by the following: (i) Any representative of the Secretary; (ii) Any representative of the State: (iii) The resident's individual physician; (iv) The State long term care ombudsman (established under section 307(a)(12) of the

Older Americans Act of 1965); (v) The agency responsible for the protection and advocacy system for developmentally disabled individuals (established under part C of the Developmental Disabilities Assistance and Bill of Rights Act); (vi) The agency responsible for the protection and advocacy system for mentally ill individuals (established under the Protection and Advocacy for Mentally Ill Individuals Act); (vii) Subject to the resident's right to deny or withdraw consent at any time, immediate family or other relatives of the resident; and (viii) Subject to reasonable restrictions and the resident's right to deny or withdraw consent at any time, others who are visiting with the consent of the resident.

(2) The facility must provide reasonable access to any resident by any entity or individual that provides health, social, legal, or other services to the resident, subject to the resident's right to deny or withdraw consent at any time.

(3) The facility must allow representatives of the State Ombudsman, described in paragraph (j)(1)(iv) of this section, to examine a resident's clinical records with the permission of the resident or the resident's legal representative, and consistent with State law.

(k) **Telephone.**

The resident has the right to have reasonable access to the use of a telephone where calls can be made without being overheard.

(l) **Personal property.**

The resident has the right to retain and use personal possessions, including some furnishings, and appropriate clothing, as space permits, unless to do so would infringe upon the rights or health and safety of other residents.

(m) **Married couples.**

The resident has the right to share a room with his or her spouse when married residents live in the same facility and both spouses consent to the arrangement.

(n) **Self-Administration of Drugs.**

An individual resident may selfadminister drugs if the interdisciplinary team, as defined by § 483.20(d)(2)(ii), has

determined that this practice is safe.

(o) **Refusal of certain transfers.**

(1) An individual has the right to refuse a transfer to another room within the institution, if the purpose of the transfer is to relocate — (i) A resident of a SNF from the distinct part of the institution that is a SNF to a part of the institution that is not a SNF, or (ii) A resident of a NF from the distinct part of the institution that is a NF to a distinct part of the institution that is a SNF.

(2) A resident's exercise of the right to refuse transfer under paragraph (o)(1) of this section does not affect the individual's eligibility or entitlement to Medicare or Medicaid benefits. [56 FR 48867, Sept. 26, 1991, as amended at 57 FR 8202, Mar. 6, 1992; 57 FR 43924, Sept. 23, 1992; 57 FR 53587, Nov. 12, 1992; 60 FR 33293, June 27, 1995]

www.ingramcontent.com/pod-product-compliance
Lightning Source LLC
Chambersburg PA
CBHW071000040426
42443CB00007B/592